I DID IT!

Acquire Skills to Change Your Life and Body

Salam S. Hachem, RD, NCSF, AFAA

BALBOA.
PRESS
A DIVISION OF HAY HOUSE

Balboa Press books may be ordered through booksellers or by contacting:

Balboa Press
A Division of Hay House
1663 Liberty Drive
Bloomington, IN 47403
www.balboapress.com
1 (877) 407-4847

Print information available on the last page.

ISBN: 978-1-5043-4924-6 (sc)
ISBN: 978-1-5043-4926-0 (hc)
ISBN: 978-1-5043-4925-3 (e)

Library of Congress Control Number: 2016902055

Balboa Press rev. date: 06/14/2016

Take your time to respond to the questions asked in this book. Be objective and most importantly be fair to yourself. In most situations, getting emotional will keep you further from results and your genuine intentions

I have known Salam for all my life and had the pleasure to work beside her and view her care towards health. This book comes at a time that is very much needed to go back to the basics and reevaluate our behavior and learning towards health.

Salam has over 25 years in the Health and fitness industry and has effected many lives and given hope to many people to find it with in themselves to be healthy and fit.

Faye Sibai, Personal Trainer

To my amazing daughter, Hala, for her constant support, love, and unending belief in me. What you have given me is immeasurable. Hala, I thank you sincerely.

To my husband, who accepts me for who I am and never attempts to put an end to my dreams.

To my sons, who make me proud of what and who they have become due to the journey we have shared.

Last but not least, to my mom, who relentlessly encouraged me throughout my life, every step of the way.

Table of Contents

Preface xi

Acknowledgments...xv

Introduction...xvii

1. About You.. 1

2. Defining a Successful Dieter.............................5

3. How to Use This Book....................................9

4. Your Action, Your Change.............................11

5. The ABCs of Behavior 13

6. Strategies.. 19

7. Nutrition 101 55

8. Checklist.. 61

9. Helpful Hints 63

10. Meal Plans..67

11. Recipes 69

Preface

I have been blessed to touch many lives in many different, positive ways. My inspiration comes from my personal and professional experiences. My gratification is the ongoing success my clients and health club members continue to experience as we learn and experiment in this ongoing process. Hence, I am included in this journey.

A nutritional, physical, and emotional state of mind has always intrigued me and has played a major part in my life on many levels. A year after I graduated in Dietetics and Nutrition from the university, my son, who was eighteen months at the time, was diagnosed with type I diabetes. He is now twenty-seven years old. Three years ago, he was diagnosed with thyroid cancer and required a complete thyroid removal. Two days prior to his thyroid surgery, he had his wisdom teeth removed. When the dental assistant informed me the procedure was complete, and my son was ready to go home, I remember his confused and worried look. Apparently, the dental assistant had shared her experience with him regarding her thyroid cancer. She mentioned how it caused her weight gain, lack of energy, and depression due to hormone imbalance.

As we stepped into the parking lot, my son said, "Mom, I am so scared I am going to be like her."

"This is a choice you make," I replied. "You need to recognize that it will be difficult until your body adjusts, but do not allow yourself to rationalize laziness or change of your eating habits because of removal of your thyroid."

Since then, he has competed in over fifty Spartan races, in addition to twice running fifty miles through Nicaragua's volcano.

About seven years ago, I was diagnosed with Hashimoto's disease. Hashimoto's often leads to an underactive thyroid gland (hypothyroidism), which leads to weight gain, lethargy, hair loss, and brittle nails. Like my son, I must take Synthroid—a replacement for a hormone normally produced by your thyroid gland—every day for the rest of my life. My son and I chose not to use the disease as a reason to be overweight and unhealthy.

I have heard about the thirty, forty, or more pounds women put on postpartum. When I ask how old their children are, they often respond that their kids are in college. Women sometimes feel entitled to gain weight during pregnancy but then keep it on postpartum. My four kids are a blessing, and I never felt the need to put on excess pounds during or after pregnancy.

There seems to be so much talk about not eating past a certain time in the evening. It is not ideal to continue to eat late in the evening in addition to your dinner. If you have a reasonable dinner, it's best not to then gorge on comfort food laden with carbohydrates, sugar, and fat before going to bed.

Snacking before you sleep can help keep your metabolism working and stabilize blood sugar levels during the night, but the recommended pre-bedtime snack is around 200–300 calories, mainly protein and no simple carbohydrates. At one point in my career, I worked the evening shift at the hospital and got home at ten o'clock at night. I can assure you I did not go to bed on an empty stomach, but I ate sensibly.

This book is not the answer to why some people lose weight and others do not. It is not the final answer to fixing an unhealthy lifestyle or behavior. It is a book of strategies geared to the individual; it's a complete lifestyle makeover. You will actively write your personal ideas and therefore become aware of what has prevented you from being mentally and physically healthy.

The strategies offered in this book will assist you in recognizing behaviors and raise awareness that will be conducive to your overall success. Strategies are not limited to dietary habits and formulating a meal plan. You will be able to relate the strategies to the different parts of your life.

Acknowledgments

I appreciate and thank my health club members and clients who have encouraged and accepted me for my convictions. You have understood my passion for educating and assisting you in your health journey.

A special thanks to Gladys and Hala, who helped with the recipes and the final stages of transferring recipes from paper to the kitchen.

Introduction

Although weight loss is the ultimate goal, don't get hung up on the weight factor. This book will set you on the path to making lifelong changes without compromises. The strategies, meal plan, along with delicious and easy-to-prepare recipe ideas will get you to your goal. In time, after applying the strategies, you will see a balanced you. Your energy will be channeled to a healthier you. Your body shape and weight will naturally alter, and you will recognize it is not about eating less but eating right. You will realize the scale is not indicative of your effort and hard work. Strategies will become so much a part of your life and not only for nutrition; you will adapt them to various parts of your life.

The practices described in this book will gradually become your lifestyle practices. The strategies will enable you to lose weight and maintain that weight loss. These small changes will make the biggest impact on your health and everyday living.

This is a self-improvement book—a hands-on guide—that will help you acquire skills that can be used in almost any situation or environment. Some people will want to take the easy way out; giving up becomes a comfortable and easier option. They aren't willing to take a chance on what has worked for so many, or they make excuses for why the strategies did not work, rather than what they can do to make it work.

It's easy to assume the thyroid does not function correctly or that you have a "slow metabolism." Unfortunately, those who do not succeed simply did not take the time to establish and accomplish their goals.

Is there a part of your life—physically or emotionally—that you wish you could alter? If so, then this book is for you.

1

About You

It seems as if there is a new weight-loss plan or program every day that promises to help shed pounds fast and easy. How many diets have you attempted? Some overweight people seem to have spent 85 percent of their lives on diets, and may always be hunting for the next fad diet. Yes, they are the victims of diet offers and weight-loss come-ons. The "new you" promises are so misleading that victims believe that the same technology that has repeatedly failed now will work.

Many books, magazines, and newspaper articles offer different formulas for success, providing the how-to based on the knowledge, beliefs, and experiences of professionals and nonprofessionals. If you read social media posts about food, supplements, or programs that claim to be the final answer to weight loss, you'll notice the numerous diets, supplements, and programs available.

How many diets have you attempted? One? Three? Five? Too many to count? How long did you keep the weight off? Did you feel healthy? Day to day, did it work for you or against you?

Here are just a few weight-loss diets that people have claimed worked for them—and you may have attempted yourself:

- Atkins
- Ornish (consists of fruits, vegetables, and grains)
- McDonald Diet
- Subway Diet
- Low-carb, low-glycemic, high-protein
- Cabbage Soup Diet
- Master Cleanse Diet
- Caveman Diet
- Alkaline Diet
- 3-Hour Diet
- Blood Type Diet
- Grapefruit Diet

There's even the Cookie Diet. So what is the best "diet" for you? The best diet for anyone is one that is doable for short and long term. Here are some questions to ask yourself:

- How long can I stick to this "diet"?
- How many days can I go without carbs?
- How long can I go without eating any fats?
- How much protein can I take in without abusing my body's organs?
- How long can I only eat fat and zero carbohydrates (similar to Atkins)?
- Can I manage this diet with my lifestyle, or will it interfere?

If you have any doubt regarding your responses, the diet is not doable, and definitely not for you. It is only a short-term fix if it does not address the issues that lead you to the negative behavior behind your eating habits. It is a diet, not a regimen.

Diets are a short-term fix, and once you stop the diet, you will go back to whatever you were doing before you started.

Temporarily, a diet may help you shed the weight off. However, it does not change your life because most diets will not change your *lifestyle*. When the diet is over, you still have the same habits and daily routines that initially caused the weight gain. Unless you have a medical ailment, the word *diet* should not be part of your vocabulary. Rather, consider behavior modification and lifestyle change.

How do you view yourself? Are you happy with yourself? Although you may be happy, how is your mental and physical health? Do you want to feel mentally healthy as well as physically healthy? If you don't start today, where do you see yourself in the next couple of months? Are you gaining, maintaining or losing weight? If your response is gaining or maintaining weight and your goal is to lose, then there is no better time to start than *now*.

Don't assume past weight losses and gains hinder your present or future attempts. It does not matter how many times you've lost and regained the weight; shedding pounds is good for your health and total well-being any time. In fact, your body will be prepared to handle the healthier change quickly.

Many people encounter barriers—personal, social, or environmental factors that vary from person to person—to maintaining their commitment to new, healthy behavioral changes. Did you lose weight and gain it back? Why did you regain the weight? Which factors contributed to the weight gain? For the most part, it may be that you reverted to old habits. People become complacent and less aware of the habits that assisted them in becoming healthy. On the other hand, if you become mindless about some strategies but maintain others, you more than likely will not get frustrated; you will be able and willing to channel your energy back into the positive behavior and get back on track.

List three reasons why you feel the need to get healthy and fit. Be specific.

1.

2.

3.

Whenever you go astray from your commitments and goals, review your reasons and analyze the importance of your new health plan.

2

Defining a Successful Dieter

Defining your success by the number on the scale is not reasonable or practical. I recommend you weigh yourself every two weeks, and do so in the morning before eating and working out. Getting on the scale daily may deter you, as it does not show your physical and mental improvement.

There are several reasons your scale may not move in your favor. For example, your weight may fluctuate due to water retention or constipation, consumption of extra salt, or insufficient water intake (dehydration).

Perseverance is the key during a setback, and the scale may create a setback if it does not show weight loss. Why assume you are not getting results, despite your hard work, if the scale does not pop up the number you were aiming to achieve. Instead, a measuring tape, body mass index, body fat analyzer, or blood work is a good way to monitor and record your progress.

For your fitness level, you can measure heart rate by doing a pulse check or using a heart-rate monitor. Heart-rate monitors are inexpensive, user-friendly, and great tracking devices. Also, time and distance can be used to measure improvement for your cardiovascular conditioning. Account for every extra minute you walk, run or use a cardiovascular equipment. Increasing your cardio time or distance is an indication you are increasing your endurance and stamina. These methods can cost close to nothing and can be done at home or gym.

Success is not only defined by achieving your ideal body weight (IBW) or goal weight (GW). During every nutritional consultation, I ask the question, "What is your goal weight?" I am never surprised by the response, "I used to weigh _____" You will achieve success when you opt for and routinely practice healthier choices—at which point it will become part of your lifestyle and will be an ongoing process. Naturally, you will make healthier choices without having to think about it.

Temporary changes in eating create temporary weight-loss results. The assumption is that we should remove old habits, rather than replacing them with better habits. For example, many of us do very well during the week, but on the weekend we eat out and blow the so-called diet. For many of us, it may not feasible to stop eating out, so a better approach is to make better choices in restaurants that cater to our new healthy well-being. Do a little research before dining out. Most chains list nutrition information online. A little homework will help you make healthy decisions that complement your new healthy lifestyle.

Find healthy foods you enjoy. Try new foods. If you did not grow up loving fruits or vegetables, there is still hope. Continue to try the food and eventually you may lose the aversion to it. Nevertheless, if Brussels sprouts, broccoli, or celery is not on top of your list, try a different green.

What makes some people successful at losing weight and keeping it off while others are unsuccessful? Successful dieters adhere to a lifestyle that includes a meal plan that is not restrictive but is part of their daily regimen. Consciously or subconsciously, the successful person answered the question of why he or she wanted to be healthy, fit, and lose weight, and finally, that person decided to commit to the goals and results he or she sought. Fit and healthy outweigh the plate of pasta or the ganache cake.

Doing the smallest thing that is good for your mind and body will help you stay on track. This will provide you with confidence and encouragement to persist in this lifelong journey. Motivation drives success. What is your motivation?

The successful dieter stays on point with a positive attitude and a can-do mind-set. Focus on the outcome and not the challenges along the way. For example, you may like to travel but not the time spent flying. For me to travel home is about a fourteen-hour flight. If I focused on the actual flight, layover, delays, finding my luggage, and anything that might go wrong, I would never take the trip. Therefore, I focus on the outcome. I envision landing at the airport and the happy faces waiting for their loved one. It helps me to get through the flight with flying colors.

After a rigorous workout, which you thought you would never finish, you say *I did it!*

Saying no to your favorite pizza or ice cream gives you a feeling of control—*I said no! I did it!* Similarly, when you feel exhausted yet convince yourself to go to the gym, you may end up with one of the best workouts you have ever had. Afterward, you again have the feeling of *I did it!*

3

How to Use This Book

I have collected a slew of simple, practical strategies to safeguard healthy behavior. They can be applied at any time, anywhere, and in any situation. Take every opportunity to implement these strategies into your daily life, and practice them, even if it does not pertain to food.

Consider these strategies as a pick-and-choose list. And whatever you do, don't give up! How many times did you attempt to ride a bicycle? When you fell, you got up and tried again, and every attempt became easier. Treat your past unsuccessful experiences as an experiment. By assuming they were failures, you are setting yourself up for another one. Do not allow past failures to define the person you can and will become. Embrace the opportunity to grow, learn, and move forward.

Understanding, learning, and practicing will be key to your success. Practice does not make you perfect; perfecting your practice at any level will make you perfect.

Take your time to respond to the questions asked in this book. Be objective and, most important, be fair to yourself. Like many situations, getting emotional will keep you farther from results and your genuine intentions.

4

Your Action, Your Change

The smallest action that leads to change may be a challenge, yet will help you to achieve results and your desired outcome. On the other hand, what you ingest could stall your progress, whether "bad" or possibly "good" food. If overindulging in good food causes you to feel guilty and puts negative thoughts in your head, those guilty feelings may stop you from reaching your intended goal. You need to possess a desire to change and act on it. You need to genuinely feel and verbalize you are ready to be fit and healthy. If your actions, which are your choices, are contrary, positive change will *not* occur.

Just because your spouse, children, family, or friends would like you to make a change is not enough. No change will be made if you don't believe, feel the need, and want to change. You need to want results. You achieve results from positive action and then positive change will happen. As challenging as it may be, do not give up. Consistently remind yourself you are doing great. The strategies are intended to improve your actions, even in a moment of despair. Do not put yourself down because of one or two negative actions you took. Rather, reinforce the small positive steps you took to prevent a full-blown mishap. Acknowledging the misstep is s positive action, which can lead to future positive and permanent change.

So many people have done it before you. The young, the old, the healthy, and the not so healthy. Consider yourself next in line.

No matter how miniscule the change is, it matters, and it will give you the motivation to make changes that are significant.

Change your mind, and your life will change!

What are three actions you will take to move toward a successful you?

1.

2.

3.

Once you take action, what will the outcome be?

1.

2.

3

5

The ABCs of Behavior

As you proceed with your journey, you will learn ways to strategize behavior to be mindfully healthy. You may become careless or mindless in one or more strategies, but continue to adhere to others that will assist you. We will use the ABC approach. ABC stands for antecedents, behavior, and consequences. These usually occur together in a series of steps called the "behavioral chain."

Antecedents are feelings and situations that occur *before* any event. For example, how do you feel emotionally and physically before eating or working out?

Behavior refers to *related* events and feelings. In reference to eating, think about speed of eating, rate of chewing, taste of food, feeling satisfied or extremely full, or any event during the process. In respect to working out, consider the time, intensity, and the type of workout. What are some sabotage strategies you use in order not to workout? What behavior will you take to prevent this from happening? For example, after work it gets difficult to convince yourself to go home and then hit the gym. A reasonable behavior would be to take your workout clothes with you and not go home but straight to the gym.

Consequences are feelings and attitude that *follow* an event. Evaluating the aftermath of your actions and awareness of the antecedent that led to the behavior are factors that can help determine if change must be made for improvement to occur. For example, after a long, hard day at work, you get home and ravage the pantry or refrigerator. You do this without being fully aware of your action. When you become thoughtless, you do not realize the type and amount of food you consume. In that moment, stop to recognize if you are emotionally or physically hungry. Those actions are your antecedents. Losing your thought of what and how much goes in your mouth is your negative behavior. On the other hand, stopping the all-out marathon on how much you are eating is your positive behavior. Once you become mindful, guilt sets in for indulging—that's the negative consequence. However, if you stop when you felt that you could have continued, is your positive consequence.

What if you are mindful and aware of what you do once you are home? You take a couple of minutes to unwind. You don't do anything that may add stress, like opening mail or reading your e-mail. Your antecedent is acknowledging your tired feelings will not go away by irrational eating or drinking. What if you took off your work clothes and changed into something that makes you feel fresh, comfortable, and just plain good? What if you did some stretches, brushed your teeth, went for a brisk walk, watered your plants, or walked the dog. Taking time to prepare your meal and not adding eight hundred calories to your evening via food tasting is your behavior. Feeling great about what and how you took care of yourself by staying in tune with your body by using the ABCs is the great feeling of consequences.

What are three things you can do to unwind before eating?

1.

2.

3.

Reflect how great you feel when you are in control, not only of what you eat but staying away from what you chose not to eat.

Listen to your body. Practice, and see for yourself what an amazing feeling it is to be in control of your actions that will invoke your change. Every time you practice this skill, it becomes easier to walk away from the table or food that may jeopardize your result. Think about the antecedents that occur before eating. Are you feeling stressed? Are you emotionally hungry? Are you happy or sad?

When these feelings occur prior to eating, how does it affect your overall eating pattern? Which emotion causes you to eat more or eat less?

- Stressed—I eat more or less?
- Hungry—I eat more or less?
- Happy—I eat more or less?
- Sad—I eat more or less?

Stress has been associated with emotional eating. To comfort ourselves, we turn to food. Afterward, the original emotional issue remains, yet we also feel worse for using food as relief. We need to realize the situations that caused our stress will not diminish by eating or drinking. On the contrary, it will only increase our stress levels and decrease confidence.

There is a difference between physical and emotional *hunger*. Physical hunger allows you to recognize when you are satisfied, at which point you stop eating. If you continue to eat beyond satisfaction, it is emotional hunger, and you are ignoring the antecedent.

Being happy does not entitle you to overeat. Celebrate your happiness as you celebrate your healthy mind and healthy body. You will have a sense of happiness if you achieve your desired goal. Assume you are at a party, and you consume fewer alcoholic beverages than usual, or maybe you do not drink at all. You may have passed on the hors d'oeuvres or not had seconds. Consequently, you are happy and have a feeling of self-accomplishment.

On the other hand, doing the opposite will set you back emotionally and have no benefits to your intended goal. Sad emotions and feelings will not disappear by eating them away. You will only increase those emotions by eating senselessly.

Can you think of three negative antecedents you have a habit of doing that you must change in order to feel better?
1.
2.
3.

Name three things you can do to de-stress? Eating is not an option!
1.
2.
3.

Can you visualize yourself doing the above? Yes or no?

Apply the ABCs to physical activity that is not a planned exercise routine. For example, if you have stairs available to you, ABC is used:
A. Point out where you have stairs available to you.
B. Go up the stairs.
C. Feel great, healthy, and energized.

Behavior sets a precedent to habits. Ultimately, it determines how likely goals are achieved. Be mindful to embellish positive behavior in order to increase the likelihood of your success.

Consequences—the end result of behavior—can either increase or diminish confidence and self-esteem.

6

Strategies

Webster's Dictionary defines *strategy* a careful plan or method for achieving a particular goal, usually over a long period; it's the skill of making or carrying out plans to achieve a goal.

What are your health goals? If your answer is to be healthy and fit, physically and emotionally, then you are in luck. The following strategies are uncomplicated and doable. Success will be achieved once you commit. Become aware, understand, and execute the strategies; this will define and drive your behavior to succeed. The strategies provided will allow you to form the foundation for success, not only for weight loss but also for maintaining healthy habits. Consider them self-management for your daily life. Adhering to them will prevent interference with your progress. Start by picking two or three strategies, and work your way from there. Do not attempt to work on all strategies at once. You will discover and experience that they are inter-related.

Apps

There are countless fitness devices and apps to help track calories in and calorie out, such as myfitnesspal.com, Lose It., Calorie Counter, Diet Tracker, and My Diet Coach—Weight Loss, to name a few. These aps are free and easy to use. You will learn quickly how the calories from snacking add up and how much exercise is needed to lose extra calories or create a deficit for weight loss. The website fitday.com is a free service—you can post online and get assistance.

Apps are a significant motivator for eating well and exercising. Apps will assist you in awareness of what and how much you consume. On any given day, if calories are higher than they should be, you can create a deficit by eating less, exercising more or both.

Review and download apps available on your smartphone, iPad, or computer. The app should be appealing and user-friendly to you.

Which app did you download?

Awareness and Being Alert

Awareness of your psychological and physical state is crucial. Awareness is a state of knowing. Being alert is the state of being watchful or attentive to present circumstances. We all "know," but are we attentive in taking the extra steps to be healthy? Think back on a conversation you might have had regarding weight loss or an exercise program. You might have an idea of what to do, but are you doing it? The goal is self-awareness and self-alertness. This will allow you to recognize your actions. Eat or don't eat; exercise or don't exercise. Are you hungry or bored? You can pick any bad food item and begin bingeing. The person who is aware and alert will stop when he or she notices a state of emotional eating. He or she will be aware of the consequences that follow. Awareness and being alert are associated with antecedent on the behavioral chain.

When your body asks for pizza or a double-fudge sundae, what it wants is not necessarily what you need. If two Oreos equal one serving, having two servings may not be too bad, but the first Oreo will taste no different from the second, fourth, or tenth. Your taste buds become immune to the real taste and flavor. If you overeat, however, do not beat yourself up. Associating food with negative or guilty emotions can escalate.

When you are aware and alert, you will be able to stop the disaster before it happens. The action and change instituted with your awareness is greater than you know, yet the results are obvious and plenty.

Active

My definition of active is not the same as working out or exercise. You might commit to a sixty-minute workout yet spend the rest of the day immobile. Active is being mindful of taking extra steps, at which point you will be on your way to a healthier and more energized lifestyle. As of today, every active action you take is a step forward to feeling invigorated. Stay in motion, not motionless. Do jumping jacks or jump squats when waiting for the shower to get hot. While brushing your teeth, do lunges or calf raises. When driving, while on your computer, or when doing dishes, tighten your abs. Park far away from your destination and walk—or run to and from your car whenever possible. In between tasks like rebooting your computer, waiting for copies, or heating your meal, do wall planks or stretches. Before using the commode, do ten squats. Whatever your job is, incorporate a couple of minutes to be physically active.

Stand often and set less. If you have a job where you sit most of the day, get out of your chair and walk around every fifteen minutes—and get water, not sugary drinks from the vending machine.

Considering your daily job routine, how can you incorporate healthy habits? Write down three things you can include daily in your job.

1.

2.

3.

Daily, before my shower, I jump rope one hundred times. If I have time, I will do another fifty or a hundred after my shower. It has made a difference in my morning attitude and energy before I head out. Purposely, I leave a magazine, keys, or any item upstairs, so I am always moving at home. For every ten steps up, you burn an average of a calorie and half—and that can reap benefits.

Day to day, how can you increase your activity level? Name three activities you will incorporate in your regular day-to-day activities.

1.

2.

3.

Balance

Balance is not only learning how to balance your "energy in" and "energy out." You need to balance your macronutrients—protein, fat, and carbohydrates. Skip the cheese, if your salad includes the allotted protein required for that meal. If the salad includes olives and chicken, you may need to skip the avocado. If you want to make a salad that includes all the array of color and flavors, you can, but each ingredient should not be a full-serving size. If you are eating a sweet potato, skip the starchy vegetable, rice, pasta, and bread.

Balance your calories daily and weekly. If you have a high calorie meal, create a deficit in the following meal. If your total daily calories are higher than your goal, balance calories the following day. Increase your exercise calorie expenditure when you have an event. This empowers you to feel dedicated but should not excuse over indulgence.

Calories

Cut back on liquid calories. Soda, fruit juice, energy drinks, sports drinks, sugary coffee drinks, and alcohol are high in sugar and have no nutritional value.

3,500 calories make one pound. A 3,500-calorie deficit will make one-pound difference for your weight loss. By eating less and working out, you will achieve this weight loss. Over time, for every 3,500 calories you take in excess, you gain one pound.

Change

Under any normal circumstances, to change you must challenge yourself. In the past, when you stagnated, did any change occur in what you attempted? You do *not* need to change your life completely to meet your health and fitness expectations. Consistency, time, and adding strategies one at a time—can add up. At which point change will happen. The smallest change can achieve great results.

> "The secret of change is to focus all of your
> energy not on fighting the old,
> but on building the new."
> —Socrates

Control

On a day-to-day basis, you control many parts of your life. You tend to overlook productivity when tasks and actions become a habit. It's unfortunate, people with weight issues often assume they have no self-control.

The same way you control and use restraint in one part of your life, apply it to your health and well-being. Write down as many things as you can think of that you do control. For example, you control waking the kids and making sure they get breakfast and get to school on time; you control getting to work on time. You also have control over something as small as not getting upset if someone takes your parking space, not losing your cool when your kid spits up on your favorite sweater, telemarketers that refuse to stop calling, or bad drivers.

However you apply control in one situation, apply it to what you choose to eat or not eat. Periodically remind yourself of goals you have set, which will promote self-control by preventing discouragement.

Take a deep breath and learn to relax. You cannot sit at the dinner table and assume you can control what goes in your mouth if you are anxious, tired, or stressed. Before heading into a meeting, *visualize* yourself with the control and confidence you will need to address issues, and, more important, control emotional eating before, after or during your meeting.

Short bouts of moderate intense exercise can boost self-control. You can control when, how, and the type of workouts you do—this requires self-restraint and control. Eventually, you learn to simulate the same control to other parts of your life.

Practice, practice, and practice to control parts of your life that inhibit you from achievement, which will assist you in maintaining a successful cycle. If you have a habit of eating your kids' leftovers or tasting the food you serve others, become mindful and take control of your actions. Be mindful and change the action that may be challenging but will provide you the control you need to succeed.

Cravings

In order to understand and resolve cravings, you must be aware of the occurrence—be *attentive* of what triggers your cravings. Once you identify the trigger food or situation, you will be able to control cravings. Environmental factors can determine if your craving will occur and to what extent. Therefore, if you control your environment, your craving will be controlled.

Exercise has proven to reduce cravings, but there's no need to head to the gym when a craving hits. Simply take a walk or do anything physical—you will be less likely to cave in to the craving, or it may not be as intense.

Identify your craving if it is for sweets, sour or salt. Substitute for a healthier choice. If sweets you want, eat raisins, dates, banana and peanut butter, semi-sweet chocolate or any fruit preserves on Ezekiel bread. I have included a recipe that is low in fat and calorie, high in protein and will sure satisfy your sweet tooth.

If you are craving sour, eat lemon with a dash of salt, pickles, carrots sticks with lime and dash of salt and pepper, or granny smith apples.

If you crave salt, have the multi-grain crackers by Crunchmaster, fat-free popcorn, or any of the baked chips available in your super market. This is only to satisfy a craving but not to do daily. Once you have the serving of your craving, brush your teeth, drink water, or eat a mint to reduce or take away the flavor your craving.

Should you give in to your sinful craving, have a little of the bad and more of the good food. For example, if you are craving ice cream, get the serving, but instead of the high-fat toppings, add fruits or nuts. You will end up eating less of the bad and more of the good. Reinvent your favorite not-so-healthy craving. If you like hamburgers and pizza, make a healthy version. It may take time to get used to, but eventually you will get the hang of it.

By not caving in to cravings, you are making a choice, not a sacrifice.

Discipline

Lack of discipline may be one of the biggest problems people encounter. Discipline is doing what you need to do whether you want to or not. Discipline requires motivation and motivation drives success. Once discipline is established and motivation is lost, discipline will keep you on point.

Consider self- discipline as a positive endeavor, rather than a punishment. Schedule yourself to drink water, work out, eat your meals, grocery shop, use stairs, park your car far, get out of your seat every fifteen minutes, do one minute or more physical activity in the morning. Eventually, you do not need to schedule it. It becomes second nature.

What are three of your motivations for getting healthy?
1.
2.
3.

What are three disciplinary actions you need to schedule throughout the day?
1.
2.
3.

Whenever you start lacking discipline, revisit your motivations written above.

Discipline may not always be an easy task, so make it fun. First, remove barriers. It is hard to push yourself to have discipline if you hate doing something. If you have trouble including exercise in your day due to time constraints, exercise for ten minutes or use the HIIT (high-intensity interval training) method. You may prefer to take classes in a group setting or do videos at home.

To be healthy, you need to be *mindfully* disciplined in your eating. This should not include eating meals you do not enjoy. Find healthy foods you do enjoy. If cooking does not come easy for you, look into having healthy meals delivered.

How many times have you said, "This is it! I am going to get healthy and fit"—and you did not. Eventually, this can lead to more of the same—failure. This happens because you form a mind-set that you don't have the necessary discipline to follow through with it.

Whenever you fall off the health wagon, what should you do? Forgive yourself. Forgive yourself, and move on. You are not perfect.

A perfectionist admits to what needs to be addressed and proceeds to work on perfecting the task. Standards for perfection vary from person to person. Therefore, work your way up from your standard base and continue working to perfect the skill—that will make you disciplined.

You could be on point most of the time and occasionally mess up. This does not mean you don't have the discipline. Like falling off your bike, you get up, dust yourself off, get back on, and start peddling.

Distraction

You may be surprised by the simple things you can do to distract yourself when you feel emotional hunger. *Distraction* does work. Try an activity that involves mind, body, or both. If you find yourself bored, sad or stressed and suddenly hungry- get busy. Go for a walk, polish your nails, call or visit a friend, web surf, play with your cat or dog, do yoga stretches, jump rope, exercise, nap, dance, or do a ten-minute workout. The following strategies are also used to avoid cravings.

At times, you may use eating or drinking as a method to distract yourself from the immediate issue at hand. Be *aware* of how you feel at that moment, and use distraction to your healthy advantage.

Downsize

The trick to losing and managing your weight is to eat less, but you should not have to experience hunger or deprivation. The key to cutting back portions and calories is to take baby steps. In several days or weeks, you will notice you need less food to hit the spot.

People gauge portions by visual cues and plate size. Increased portions lead to increased eating, which leads to weight gain. Weight gain is due to eating more because you have a larger portion of food.

The average adult consumes about 95 percent of what is on his plate. Reducing the amount you serve yourself is a good start. You will eat smaller portions by downsizing your serving plate. Practice using smaller utensils, plates, and cups. It will lead to a habit of having a smaller quantity of food. Consider the following tips:

- Remove large dishes from your environment.
- Become familiar with appropriate serving sizes by using a scale, measuring cups and spoons.
- Read food labels.
- Don't leave your cooked meal on the counter or table in front of you. Instead, serve it on the stovetop and put the extra away. Out of sight, out of mind.
- Use the serving size recommended on the package label for snacks.
- Don't eat out of the box. Take out a serving, and put away the box.
- Opt for single-serving treats.

Have you decided which utensils, plates, and cups you will use? If not, take time to do so now.

Emotional Eating

We often use the term *emotional eater* for the weak or desperate. Whether we recognize it or not, most of us with weight issues practice emotional eating. From early on, we were given food or treats when we were feeling happy, sad, or depressed. Treats were given for good grades or good behavior. Subconsciously, food is thought of as a reward or medicine. When stressed, the brain is trained to look for ways to make that bad feeling go away. You resort to what made you feel better in the past.

Unstable emotions can lead to unhealthy behavior, which leads to unhealthy habit. Your state of mind affects your relationship with food, as do many events that happen to you. Your all-around positive attitude will empower you to have better health.

Avoiding what you are emotionally feeling or experiencing can be detrimental. Emotional eating can cause your original negative state to diminish but only for the moment. To avoid negative feelings, we distract ourselves with food, eating, drinking, smoking and other behavior that keeps us preoccupied, physically and emotionally. These behaviors reduce our confidence and state of well-being. Ultimately, emotional eating can exacerbate the original issue at hand and lessen your inner strength.

When and if this does occur, *stop*. Ask yourself what you learned from this mishap. How are you smarter? Next time, how would you do it differently? You learn to recognize your trigger points, and develop a strategic plan to avoid emotional eating. Be mindful and use the ABC to recognize triggers and what happens after the fact. This will allow you to strategize the next episode.

Environmental Control (EC)

We rely on environmental triggers much more than we realize. Environmental control (EC) is an important factor in healthy well-being. When you have adequate EC, you control temptation; when you control temptation, you control intake; when you control intake, you control your weight. It is easier not to mess up if your environment is controlled.

Don't bring the wrong foods into your environment and use kids, husband, family, friends, or colleagues as an excuse. The kids and everyone else can do without the potato chips, ice cream, chocolate chip cookies, or any of *your* trigger foods. If you do not bring in the wrong foods into your environment, no one will miss those foods but you. Challenging yourself not to eat the food if it's in your environment will make you feel deprived. Deprivation will cause you to overeat other foods.

Make a list of the foods on your meal plan. When you do your grocery shopping, buy only what is on the list. What you put in your grocery cart and take home becomes the food in your environment.

At the workplace, do not go where the wrong foods are. Have your healthy snacks available at all times. Keep snacks handy so you are not tempted to visit the vending machine. Control your environment; don't let it control you. When you have environmental control, you can better control your willpower. You will fall into the habit of grabbing what is available and within reach. If sweets and fatty snacks are all you have, then that is what you will grab. If your environment has fruits, nuts, and yogurts, your only option will be to reach for healthier choices.

Water and physical activity are also factors that complement your environment. Always have water available and in front of you. Having water visible reminds you to drink. It also establishes a feeling of accomplishment to fulfill your goal on the amount you aim to drink. A feeling of, *I did it!*

Physical activity is one of the strategies mentioned earlier. Keep a jump rope, sneakers, weights, workout clothes, or anything else needed for working out in plain sight.

Be around like-minded people. Some people feel that trying every restaurant in town is a way to give themselves a reward. Reconsider your relationship with those people. The people with whom you eat may influence how much and the type of food you eat.

When dining out, be the first person to order. This will set a precedent of ordering the healthy options. You are more likely to order fried, high-fat meals if the person ahead of you places an order for curly fries with cheese and gravy.

If your commute takes you past fast-food establishments, find a different route.

During holidays or any special event, following the factors mentioned will keep you in control of a healthier environment. You may not be able to dodge all your indulgences, but you can reduce the exposure.

Excuses

Excuses are the nails used to build a house of failure.
—Don Wilder

Excuses are not reasons rather a way to rationalize and justify not committing to or pursuing goals. Instead of channeling your energy on negative excuses and knowing the results are bleak; put your energy on working towards your commitment and positive results. Excuses translates into *failure*.

Focus on all the reasons why you must achieve your goals. Once you stop making excuses, what will the outcome be? Achieving results is a valid reason to stop making excuses and that translates into *success*. A feeling of *I did it!*

Name three excuses you have used that will not help you achieve your health and fitness goals.

1.

2.

3.

Review your excuses and determine their validity. Write a resolution for every excuse.

1.

2.

3.

Exercise

It's clear, most of us may not like or appreciate strenuous exercise. This is comparable to people who have little appreciation for brushing or flossing their teeth. You know the benefits of brushing and flossing, and the outcome if you don't.

The "perfect" exercise is the one you are happiest doing. Consider your workout time as a break—a well-earned and deserved break. Every one of us deserves "*me*" time. People have the tendency to eat less when they work out for emotional rather than physical reasons.

On average, every minute you walk extends your life by one and a half to two minutes.

Time—or lack of it—is the number-one reason people claim they can't exercise. Non-exercisers have as much time as exercisers—that is, everyone has twenty-four hours in the day. Figure out a way to schedule exercise daily. Start with a morning or afternoon walk. Start with a commitment to ten minutes a day and work your way up.

Short interval training replaced the hour-plus cardio sessions. HIIT classes and Tabatha trainings are all over the gyms and internet. These are high intense short burst workouts. Use the fitness app you downloaded to monitor your progress.

Exercise achieves a post-workout calorie burn and post-workout high—it's a feeling of *"I did it!"*. Trigger food cannot give you that.

If you decide to join a gym, consider the proximity to your job, school, or home. Ideally, the gym should be on your way to work, school, or home or in between. Get a feel for the gym. Review the classes offered. What are the operational hours? Is it open when you will use it most? If you have children, does the gym offer babysitting services? Will there be someone to assist you in the gym, or does the gym suggest you hire a trainer at extra cost? You should feel relaxed and not intimated while working out. I have noticed women feel more comfortable in all-women gym.

Remember that exercise generates energy, and the more energy you have, the more you accomplish.

Among other benefits, exercise can improve your emotional well-being. Ultimately, you will notice physical benefits as well. This feeling will empower you, and the number on the scale will not deter your progress if it does not change.

Saying "I'm going to start working out" is wishy-washy. Commit to the time and place you will work out. Complete the following statement:

The length of time I am willing to commit to my physical well-being is _____minutes.

Will you join a gym? Yes or No
    If yes, which gym will you join?
    If no, where will you exercise?

How many days can you commit to exercising?

Initially when you start an exercise program, your weight may not come off as fast as you hope it will, but your body fat, body mass index, and blood work will improve. Your total body inches and waistline will decrease. You will go up the stairs without gasping for air or feeling a heart attack about to come on. The commitment to exercise is an accomplishment and more rewarding than the number on the scale. Exercise gives an overall sense of accomplishment. Tracking time, exercises (reps and sets), or distance walked can be extremely motivating. Progress serves as a benchmark and helps increase your goal.

Your goal should be to build lean muscle, lose unwanted fat, increase or maintain bone density and decrease total cholesterol. It is common to see clothing size or body fat composition decrease even if your weight remains the same.

You can eat more when you decrease body fat and preserve muscle mass. A person who diets without exercising loses a combination of fat and muscle. Approximately 25 percent of total loss without exercise comes from muscle mass.

Exercise regularly. Your negative state of mind will diminish, and your positive state of mind will flourish.

Failure

It is a good idea to use trial and error when actively attempting to reach your goal. Any "diet" or exercise program you did in the past was a trial. If it did not work, it is the error you must address and correct this time around. Plan, plan, and plan some more. Planning will decrease the likelihood of failing or being blindsided. Planning will be your road map to success.

You succeed not because you don't experience failure, rather it's your commitment and perseverance that will get you there.

When faced with a disappointment, think about the positive parts in your life, along with your day-to-day accomplishments. Make a list of achievements. Nothing is too small to write down and acknowledge.

You can learn from failure if you are mindful of the action. A hundred failures from your past are not as important as one achievement today. It is never too late to start. Only you can make failure an option. Any time is a great time to start—and that's when failure fails and succeeding prevails.

Focus

Focus is power. Focus on immediate goals and the processes that go along with them. The instant gratification of achieving smaller goals will be more satisfying than looking at the bigger picture. Do not center your attention on what you are giving up. Focus on the benefits, outcome, and your success.

When you do an intense workout. if you focus on thinking, *I am going to die*, you will quit. Instead, focus on how rewarding it feels when you complete your workout, and say *"I did it."* Ultimately, you will learn to embrace the challenges along the way.

Focus on your commitment. A small decision can make the greatest difference for the rest of your day, week, month ... and maybe your life.

Food Labels

Read before you eat. This will allow you to be *mindfully aware* of what you are about to ingest. Food labels may appear confusing but are simple once you learn the basics. Food labels begin with nutrition facts:

1. Serving size—numbers are based on one serving size. The package may contain several servings. This is critical information that will assist with portion control.
2. Calories—the total calories per serving (not for the total package).

3. Total fat—the amount of the different kinds of fat in one serving, including saturated fats (not good for you heart fat) and unsaturated (good for your heart fat).
4. Cholesterol and sodium (salt)—the amount in one serving. Choose food that is low in cholesterol and sodium. Look for 5 percent or less for cholesterol per serving. Limit salt to 2,300 milligrams daily (about 1 tsp).
5. Protein—total grams per serving. High-protein foods can relatively be high in fat.
   Look for lean protein like egg whites, fish, turkey, chicken and lean red meats.
6. Percent Daily Values— based on the percent of serving for a 2,000-calorie diet. For example, if the label lists 10 percent for sodium, it means that one serving provides 10 percent of the sodium you need each day. Daily values may be higher or lower, depending on calorie requirement for the individual.

The fitness app you downloaded will assist you in keeping a food record. Reading food labels, however, will enable you to make the decision when buying the food item and bringing it in to your environment.

Freeze
Most often, frozen vegetables and fruits are as nutritious as fresh ones. Flash-frozen vegetables and fruits may contain more nutrients than out-of-season fresh produce. Vegetables and fruits harvested for freezing are processed at their peak ripeness. Fresh produce is sometimes placed for a longer time than desirable under lights on the store shelves. The continued water spraying and lighting make produce look more appealing and fresh than it actually is. A good rule of thumb is to purchase what is in season and use immediately.

There is not much difference in the amount of fiber for fresh or frozen fruits and vegetables. Always have fruits and vegetables in your freezer as an alternative. Do avoid frozen vegetable bags with heavy sauces and creams. Canned vegetables may be an option if rinsed before use or if they are labeled "low sodium."

Who said eating healthy has to be expensive? Delicious, nutritious produce does not necessarily cost a lot of money. A frozen bag of vegetables can be less than $1.25.

Spruce up your meatballs or hamburgers with extra vegetables. Spinach and mushrooms are nearly calorie-free and can go unnoticed by children when combined with ground turkey meat. Shred carrots into your favorite tomato sauce. Puree spinach and add to soup or sauces.

Vegetables are packed with vitamins. Vitamin A for eyes and skin. Vitamin C spurs the immune system and protects against cardiovascular and eye disease and wrinkles. Red and green peppers, strawberry, kiwi, tomato juice, cauliflower, Brussels sprouts, oranges and mangoes.

Vitamin E is an antioxidant that can neutralizes free radicals that can cause cell degeneration to prevent cancer. Vitamin E is found in kiwi, mangoes, tomatoes, spinach, and broccoli.

Vitamin K beneficial for blood clotting and the body's ability to repair itself. Vitamin K is found in lettuce, spinach, cabbage, string beans, and Brussels sprouts.

Vitamin B reduces heart disease and stroke, help nervous system and help break down carbohydrate. Vitamin B can be found in lentils, dark leafy vegetables, beans, berries and bananas.

Goals

Goal setting directs you toward a desired outcome. Establish your goals. Once goals have been thought out and strategized, you will know clearly where you want to go. Your goals must be clearly defined—this is similar to planning a trip, party or a work project. You are more likely to achieve your goals once you clearly establish them, and less likely to get lost in the day-to-day hustle and bustle.

True, defined goals are measurable, achievable, and attainable, which ultimately leads to your desired outcome.

If your goals are unclear or too drastic, you may give up. Give yourself a reasonable range. If you want to lose sixty pounds, start with a ten- to fifteen-pound weight loss goal.

When you start an exercise program, aim to work out three to four times per week. This is a doable goal. Do not set a goal of going to the gym seven days a week. This may be unrealistic due to time constraints—or muscle soreness. Plan how and when you will get your exercise. Will you exercise before work or after work? You may go home after work, get comfortable, and decide not to hit the gym as planned. Why not have your gym clothes in the car and head straight to the gym after work or school?

Increasing your water intake may be your goal, as it was for me a couple of years ago. Initially, my goal was to drink one liter a day. I placed the bottle on my nightstand. I got in the habit of drinking water before going to sleep, as well as before and after my shower. Initially, my goal was to drink five gulps—certainly not the whole bottle. Now, it has become a habit for me to drink much more than that.

Name three specific goals. Think achievable and measurable.
1.
2.
3.

Once you have met your goal, celebrate it. Rewards motivate and encourage you to keep going. Just remember: your reward should not be celebrating with eating and drinking. Your good feeling of accomplishment will last longer than the indulgence and is a reward in itself.

Gratitude

Practice daily gratitude. There are thousands of reasons to be grateful. Acknowledge and be grateful for the big and small things. Every time you say no to a second helping of food or make the right choice to better your well-being, realize that is enough reason to be grateful. Under normal circumstances, if usually you have three alcoholic drinks but choose to have two drinks or none, be grateful for that. Give yourself credit.

Be grateful when completing an exercise class. Sign up for a 5K run and be grateful for finishing, regardless of the time it takes you or where you place in the race. Being able to participate is gratifying. I teach a HIIT (high-intensity interval training) class in one of my gyms. I emphasize and continuously encourage members to finish one more repetition (rep) or one extra second they normally would not complete. This is a reason to be grateful. Whenever you start your day, jot down tasks to accomplish. When you complete tasks, feel grateful for completing those tasks.

I discourage anyone from comparing themselves to others. Everyone's base and standard is *different*. By setting your own standard, you will be grateful for your achievements.

Write three reasons you are grateful in this moment.
1.
2.
3.

Once you begin your healthy, fit mind and body, continue to add to this list.

Guilt

Guilty feelings for various situations can trigger emotional eating. Owning and acknowledging missteps can help you accept and move past them. Instead of beating yourself up for an off-day, be mindful of how you feel physically and mentally afterward. When you focus on your feelings rather than on the action, it can help you recognize the effects of your choices. Be *aware* and *alert* to the physical and emotional discomfort (consequence), in order to make better choices next time. Accept that you screwed up and move on.

You will feel guiltless making better meal choices, skipping dessert, fewer drinks, listening to your body when you're feeling full, going for that walk, jog or working out. The positive feelings you experience can carry you longer than feeling guilty or giving up.

Adhering to the environmental-control factors like water, physical activity, eating fruits and vegetables will lessen the guilt.

Do not forsake your workout because of guilt. The happiest person finds his or her "me time".

Do you feel guilty when you take out time for yourself?

Do the people around you make you feel guilty for your "me time," or do they encourage you to be a better you?

Habit

The smallest positive change in everyday negative habits can give your mental and physical well-being a boost.

What habit would you like to break? What's stopping you? It is amazing how people avoid breaking habits they know are bad for them because they assume they have no willpower. Habits cannot be broken through willpower alone. Breaking a habit is about creating a new attitude and retraining your automatic response system to perform new and better behavior.

The process takes mental preparation and a conscious plan to replace actions. How long does it take to adopt a new habit? Some people contend it takes twenty-one days. It could take up to sixty-days. I directed a four-week program, and my clients were able to change their habits that had prohibited them from weight loss in two weeks.

The first step to overcoming negative habit is acknowledging (*aware*) the habit that needs to be replaced. The second step is to take the decision that *you* want to replace the habit. You must see the benefits of making a change, be more desirous of new behaviors. Don't focus on what you are giving up. Focus instead on what you will gain.

Anyone who associates fond memories with certain bad habits will only stop those habits for a short period, if at all. Eventually, without a change of perception, the person will go back to a behavior that he or she associates with something pleasant.

Practice is a behavior repeated and repeated over time. Practice long enough, and positive behavior will turn into a habit.

List three healthy habits that you will include in your day for the next twenty-one days.

1.

2.

3.

Acknowledging and understanding your eating *habits* is an important tool to weight loss and maintenance. Recognize and repeat positive habits, and achieve the benefits.

Hunger

The two types of hunger we experience are physical and emotional.

Physical Hunger	Emotional Hunger
To a certain degree, can be satisfied with any type of food	A specific craving for a specific food
Comes on gradually, but can be delayed	Comes on quickly, with urgency
Feel satisfaction and no guilt	Feel guilty, bad, and doubtful
At the point of feeling full, you stop eating	You continue to eat to the point of feeling uncomfortable

Can you recall the last time you were physically hungry? The desire to eat starts with thoughts of food, and then you decide to take the plunge. Be aware and alert of your hunger state to determine whether you are physically hungry and you are not acting on urge. Rate your hunger. When you are about to eat, you should be hungry but not starving. Lack of food intake will cause your blood sugar to drop. If this occurs, you feel famished which may lead to overeating.

Your goal is to stop eating when you are comfortably full. Get in the habit of gauging your level of hunger:

1. Starving
2. Belly growling
3. Mild hunger (a power snack will do just fine—protein and complex carbohydrates)
4. Satisfied; don't need to finish your plate
5. More than satisfied; no need to continue eating
6. Stuffed and need to unzip your pants

Rate your satisfaction after each meal. This is as important as rating your initial hunger. It helps identify the amount of food you have consumed and at what point you should stop eating. You should stop eating at # 4 (satisfied), if you want to finish your meal later, do so. Acknowledging how uncomfortable you feel once you are at #6 (stuffed) will allow you to reconsider the next meal.

Emotional hunger causes mindless eating. We use food to subdue our emotions as a coping mechanism when feeling stressed, upset, angry, lonely, exhausted or bored. This is physically and emotionally unhealthy. If you find yourself doing this daily, it may be what is prohibiting you from your weight loss goals. Gauge your state of fullness, and if you are at #5, you're eating for emotional reasons. The only way is to be *aware* of your present state and what you must do to stop.

How and what will you do to recognize emotional hunger which has led to over eating?

What can you do to replace emotional eating with a positive behavior?

Several factors are known to have an effect on the choice to eat-smell, sight, taste and social setting, which bring us back to your *environment*.

Thirst may be mistaken for hunger. Therefore, it is best to quench your thirst to determine if you are experiencing dehydration or hunger.

There are no "rules" regarding hunger; simply eat when you are hungry, and stop when you're satisfied. Eat what gives you energy and makes you feel healthy inside and out.

Hydrate

Water is possibly the single most important nutrient for helping to lose weight and keep it off. I do not suggest drinking eight ounces of water eight times per day. I suggest you start from what you drink now and increase it by 50 percent. Keep a bottle on your desk and in your briefcase, purse, gym bag, and anywhere visible. Remember: *out of sight-out of mind.* In between e-mails, sip water. Set a goal before and/or after each meal to drink water. Set a goal to finish one liter or more by a certain time. Depending on your commute to work, set a goal to drink a certain amount_____. Strategies to increase water intake to incorporate in your daily routine.

At first, it may be inconvenient due to increased need to use the bathroom, but—this is good news—this means your body is letting go of all the toxic water it has been holding in. After a couple of days or a week, the trips to the bathroom will taper off. Your body will get into a perfect rhythm and you'll notice reduced appetite, a luminous complexion, better muscle tone, increased energy, and—most of all—an efficient metabolism.

After waking up, water helps to activate your organs. One glass of water before a meal helps with digestion. One glass of water before a bath helps lower blood pressure. One glass of water before bed helps to avoid stroke or heart attack.

Water suppresses the appetite naturally and helps the body metabolize stored fat, which means water helps break down fat and flush it out.

Drink water after your meal. This will cue your mind to know that eating has stopped, along with giving you a feeling of being full with less food consumption.

Flavor your water with fruits and vegetables. Experiment until you find a combination you enjoy. (I have provided a couple of ideas in the recipe section of this book.)

Drink water at different temperatures to see which you prefer to drink. Sipping from a water bottle can seem less daunting than pouring a big glass of water and forcing yourself to drink it.

The fastest route to more energy is adequate hydration. Start your engine.

How will you incorporate water into your daily activities?
1.

2.

3.

"I"
Say the following:
"I am important. I can and I will take care of myself. I can count on myself, as everyone counts on me. I have achieved goals, and I have goals. Day by day, I will build strength and learn to do things better. I am grateful I have the opportunity to take care of me. I am committed and devoted to taking care of me."

If I do not start today, where will I be in the next three months?

If I start today, where will I be in the next three months? You will be in a better and healthier place—and you will be able to say, *"I did it!"*

Jeopardize
Our bad eating habits not only jeopardize our health and well-being but potentially our children and family. If kids watch us eat when in distress, eat for emotional reasons, eat in front of the television screen, and not exercise, they will follow suit. We have a responsibility to our kids and the people around us.

Mindful or Mindless
Some of us swallow food without truly tasting it. If it was not for the peel you left on the counter, you might forget you ate the banana, never mind the cookies and the amount you consumed. Be mindful, and record what you eat and how

much. Remember to use the fitness app that does not forget what you eat once you record it.

Be mindful of your emotional and physical hunger state. If you are mindless, you will not recognize your present state. Be mindful of your stomach signaling your brain when you are *comfortably* satisfied. Be alert to rate hunger and satisfaction at the end of your meal. Being in tune will allow you to have what you want and not feel guilty.

When you are mindful, you will stop to read food labels and see if the food is worth the calories. Mindless eating is a problem when you are bored or dealing with a negative situation that turns into emotional eating.

You can improve your willpower and control food intake if you are mindful. Ultimately, this will empower you. Losing weight and getting fit is not about starving and dieting; it is about being *mindful!*

Moving

Get up and get moving! Doing this every fifteen to twenty minutes during a workday will help you focus and get more work done. For every fifteen minutes of sitting at your desk (or anywhere else, for that matter), get up and pace for one minute.

Run in place, jump rope, do jump squats, jumping jacks, or hold a plank. Walk to your colleague instead of e-mailing or calling them. In between, a set number of emails or calls get up and walk. Use stairs instead of taking the elevator. The goals you set to get moving will depend on your job and how you will incorporate into your daily routine.

How often and when do you plan on getting up and moving?

Motivation

What is your motivation? Is it the scale, reducing inches, or smaller dress size? Is your motivation decreasing your body fat and body mass index, which then decreases your health risk factors? Does playing with your kids or grandchildren and not feeling exhausted motivate you? How about increasing the time you spend on the treadmill? Do you want to decrease your blood work and lipid profile levels or maintain a healthy range? How about increasing longevity, yet having vitality.

Successful people are motivated for their own reasons. Name three reasons to get motivated for better health.

1.

2.

3.

Plan

Plan your goals, strategies, and success. It will not happen by accident. In order to have a healthy, clean environment and decrease the likelihood of trigger foods, you must have everything you need on hand. This requires grocery shopping. Grocery shopping requires planning, and planning requires time. Plan your grocery shopping for when you are not hungry, sleepy, or tired. Plan to have your next meal ready and prepared. This eliminates the guessing game. Double recipes when you cook and freeze extras, or save leftovers for the following day. Leftovers should be available at all times as a backup plan. Freezing extra food does not diminish the flavor or nutrients.

Prevent a "pig-out" by planning. Do not sabotage yourself by *not* planning. Fill in your plans for the following:

Plan your water._____

Plan your exercise._____

Plan your grocery shopping._____

Plan how you will increase your activity at work._____

Plan how you will increase your activity at home._____

Plan how you will do things differently for an event, party, or vacation._____

Plating

Plating can make a difference of the amount of calories you take in. "Plating" refers to the way you fill your plate. Fill half of your plate with colorful, non-starchy vegetables, like broccoli, bell peppers, tomatoes, spinach, and mushrooms. Eat vegetables before eating any of the protein or carbohydrates. You do this to fill on lower calorie food and consume less of the higher calorie. If you're right-handed, placing veggies on the right side of your dinner plate will get you to eat them first (and if you're left-handed, use the left side). Place your protein in the middle of the plate and carbohydrates or higher-calorie food on the bottom of your plate—bottom left for those who are right-handed, and bottom right for lefties.

Positive

Regardless of the outcome, stay positive. You can encourage and motivate yourself from positive thinking. Every negative situation has a positive side. You must be open to believing and seeing there is a positive side to any negative situation. If the scale did not move from the last time you weighed yourself, think about how fast you can move. Use your motivation factors to stay positive.

Have you noticed how Mondays are labeled on social media? Some of the posts I've read are somewhat humorous:

"If each day is a gift, I'd like to know where to return Mondays"

"Dear Monday, I want to break up. I'm seeing Tuesday and dreaming about Friday,

Sincerely, it's not me; it's you."

"It's Monday. Ewww!"

"Monday, *again!*"

"May your coffee be strong and your Monday be short."

I, however, decided to make Mondays the best day of the week. I made a list of the reasons Mondays are great. For example, "Beginnings are always nice, and Monday is the beginning of a new week." I decided to go to my gyms with a great, new positive attitude to start the day and my week. By asserting a positive attitude, you will have a clear mind to be objective.

Instead of drinking five drinks at an event, have two drinks along with your water. Tell yourself you did great—you could have had so much more, but you only had two. Don't dwell on what you could have done. Focus on what you will *do*. Keep building on it.

Positive thinking will push your body beyond what you thought was physically and mentally possible. And remember: positive people are grateful people.

Practice

Practice is done with conscious effort. Practice will become habitual if repeatedly done. Habit is an unconscious effort.

Practice for a healthier you, and healthier habits will develop. Practice attending an exercise session and being active. Practice being *mindful* of what you eat, drink, and increasing your water intake. Practice using the fitness app. Practice using stairs instead of the elevator. Practice keeping a clean environment. Practice healthy skills, and they will become habits. *Practice does not make you perfect; perfecting your practice will.*

Record Keeping

Keeping a food record is important for many reasons. Record keeping provides objectivity and eliminates guessing how much you've eaten. You will be able to review total calories for the day, week, or months, which will give you reason to continue on your plan. It may indicate you are undereating or overeating. Your body may be retaining water, or maybe you're not getting enough exercise.

Record keeping will reinforce the "4 P's"—positivity, persistence, planning, and practice.

Record keeping holds you accountable. Accountability plays a big part in your successful weight loss and maintenance. Record keeping can assist you with self-control. For many people, just knowing they have to write down what they are about to eat is a great deterrent to overeating. Record keeping can make you *aware* of emotional motivations for the food choices you make throughout the day. You may notice a pattern of the types of food you choose at a particular time.

It is best to record your intake immediately after eating—don't wait longer than fifteen minutes. Otherwise, you might forget what you ate. Continue to record intake, even when you are not exactly on point. This will help you not to mindlessly munch and may lead you to rethink second or third helpings. And what about "forgotten calories"—the ripped-off end of Cuban bread you tasted while waiting in line or samples provided at the store? And how about everything you taste while preparing meals? All those calories need to be included to your daily intake.

Use the fitness app you downloaded; it will help you stay in tune with whatever your eating for a healthier you. It's also a good tool to use when you feel out of control.

No one consistently can make healthy choices every second of the day, but make choices that help you feel better about yourself instead of choices that only drag you down.

Sabotage
People-pleasers need be extremely aware. To please others, these people will go out of their way to eat more than they normally would. They do this so others feel comfortable or maybe to receive acceptance. How many times have you been invited to eat a food, and you responded with a no—but the no sounds like yes? A person sabotaging you will be persistent and

continue to ask until you give in. This is due to your unsure no, but if you affirm your "**NO**", you will not be sabotaged—unless you allow it.

I never understood my clients when they claimed they ordered a certain food because "everyone at the table ordered it." At that point, no one had anything to do with sabotaging them; it was their choice.

Which is greater—getting acceptance from others or relearning to accept your healthier self?

Name three sabotage strategies you use or allow others to use in order not to succeed.

1.

2.

3.

What will you do to change this?

1.

2.

3.

Simplify

Simplify your life. Find every shortcut you can to accomplish chores and tasks. Purchase precut vegetables and salads. Double up on recipes so you have leftovers. Instead of buying ground turkey to make hamburgers, buy the ones already prepared to grill. Buy your chicken already deboned and skinless.

Put your energy in what is important—and nothing is more important than *you!*

Name three things you can simplify.

1.

2.

3.

Success

The key to success is having clarity. In order to sabotage your success, you might create distractions. Recognize what is essential and disregard what is not. To be successful in weight loss, it is more effective to add positive behavior than attempt to remove the unhealthy behavior.

Build on the willpower you already have—this pertains to any situation. Consider yourself a successful person. Everyone has had a taste of success. Apply the same strategy to weight loss that you used to succeed with any goal you have achieved. Acknowledge small results, and continue to build on them. Be grateful for any amount of success.

Talking

Talking to yourself may be a good thing. It helps clarify your ideas and plans. However, when you do talk to yourself, do it with objectivity, positivity, and respect.

When you turn down a food, tell yourself how good you feel for not eating it.

Before dining or a special event, talk to yourself about what you will and won't do. Say, "Just do it," followed with "*I did it.*" Say this aloud and see how good it feels.

Time

Often, I am asked how I manage my gyms, train, teach classes, give nutritional consultations, run a household with four kids and a husband, and find time for the things I love. I don't find time; I make time. By taking care of myself, I am in a better mind-set for everyone else.

When you view yourself as important, so will everyone else. Learn to give yourself time. By preparing meals for the week, you save time and money. It takes more time to eat out. You have to drive to the restaurant, wait to be seated, order your meal, wait for your meal, eat your meal, wait for the bill, pay the bill, and drive back home. Conversely, you could have stuck a turkey burger in the oven and had sautéed frozen vegetables.

Learn to *simplify*. If you do not have time for a sixty-minute workout, do a high-intensity workout for less time.

When there is determination, there is no time for procrastination!

Timing

Timing your meals will create balance in your body. In order to achieve your body-composition goals, it is important that you eat food throughout the day and balance your nutrients. Eating every three to four hours will provide your body with the necessary nutrients and energy to contend with daily activities and stress. Additionally, it will prevent hunger, which is the primary cause of overeating. I don't suggest, however, forcing food in your body if you are not hungry—this brings us back to eating out of habit and not for nutritional needs.

Triggers

Recognize and avoid your trigger food, people, events, and places. Change one trigger at a time. Record keeping will help you identify your triggers, at which point you will be better able to control your environment. Environmental control will help you in reducing triggers and the manifestation thereof.

Visualization

Use visualization to paint a mental image of how you want to feel and look. Recreate the image and feelings in your mind surrounding your goals. Practice visualization and imagery when you feel grateful, motivated, and positive. Hold on to the picture and feelings acquired at that exact time to remind yourself whenever you feel helpless.

Do not limit yourself due to unsuccessful experiences. Limitations are made within our own thoughts and beliefs. Be open-minded and daring.

7

Nutrition 101

As you are well aware, there is no one-size-fits-all for weight loss and maintenance, but knowing and understanding how nutrients work is a great start.

"Essential nutrients" are nutrients that your body cannot produce on its own or in adequate amount. In order for the body to function properly, these nutrients must be taken in from your food intake. The six essential nutrients include carbohydrates, protein, fat, vitamins, minerals, and water.

Carbohydrates
Carbohydrates provide the body with fuel and energy. This is our main source of energy for growth, everyday activities, and training. During the digestive process, complex carbohydrates are broken down into glucose. Glucose circulates in the blood and is the chief source of energy for refueling the liver and muscle, which is used up during exercise.

Carbohydrates contain four calories per gram. Natural carbohydrates are broken down into three categories: simple sugars, complex carbohydrates, and fibrous carbohydrates.

Simple sugars cause a relatively sharp rise in blood sugar, which can increase insulin and ultimately result in increased fat storage. Hence, high triglycerides levels in your blood.

Example of simple sugar includes fruit juice, candy, soda, and fat-free or sugar-free snack foods. Simple sugar should be avoided throughout the day, more importantly three to four hours before bedtime.

It may be challenging to refrain from eating simple sugars, but if you avoid sugar for fourteen days, you will feel and see the difference. Trust me on this one; your *craving* will diminish

Complex carbohydrates supply a slower, steady release of glucose into the bloodstream. Therefore, glucose from complex carbohydrates tends to draw a minimum insulin secretion and provide more sustained energy levels. Examples includes: quinoa, wheat germ, oatmeal, brown rice, grits, sweet potatoes, lima beans, lentils, and other legumes.

Fibrous carbohydrates come from plant foods like fruits and vegetables. Fiber slows the release of carbohydrates into the bloodstream. Examples include asparagus, broccoli, cabbage, cauliflower, celery, spinach, green beans, zucchini, and other salad greens. This category also is lower in calories and usually can be consumed throughout the day without limitations.

Fiber has been proven to reduce the risk of coronary heart disease, help regulate blood glucose levels, decrease cholesterol, and aid in preventing constipation.

Although fiber is a component of carbohydrates, it does not have any caloric value. The two types of fiber include *soluble* and *insoluble*. Soluble fiber aids in decreasing blood cholesterol, and insoluble assists in preventing constipation and increases satiety.

It is suggested forty percent of your total daily calories come from complex carbohydrate. For example, if your total caloric daily intake is 1800 calorie per day, multiply by 40 percent to get the total carbohydrate calories per day.

40 percent carbohydrate per day from 1800 calorie = 720 carbohydrate calories per day.

Protein

Protein makes up the structure of every cell in the body. It is specifically involved in the growth, repair, and maintenance of cells. Protein keeps muscles healthy and firm.

Protein is made up of individual organic compounds called amino acids and known to speed up your basic metabolic rate by 30 percent. Your basic metabolic rate is the speed at which the body burns calories while at complete rest. Protein-rich foods have a high *thermal effect* in your body. High thermal effect is the amount of energy your body uses above the resting metabolic rate, due to digesting protein.

Eating low-fat animal protein will help increase lean tissue and burn fat.

Protein contains four calories per gram. The best sources are eggs, fish, poultry, red meat, dairy products, nuts, seeds, and legumes like lentils and beans. What determines a healthy protein is the amount and type of fat it has. Protein is derived mainly from animal products. Red meats are high in protein, yet high in saturated fat. Since protein is not stored in the body, low-fat animal protein must be consumed three to four times per day in order to maintain a positive nitrogen balance. It's suggested you take in 1.0–1.5 grams of protein per pound of body weight per day. Every meal or snack should contain protein. This is your power meal or snack. Since protein takes longer to digest, it slows down the production of *ghrelin*. Ghrelin is a hormone that tells our brain that we are hungry.

35 percent of your total daily calories should come from lean protein sources. Egg whites are an excellent source of protein and essentially are fat-free, low-calorie food.

35 percent protein per day from 1800 kcal per day= 630 kcal from protein per day

Fat

Fat is an energy source when consumed increases the absorption of fat-soluble vitamins A, D, E, and K. Fat is the most concentrated source of energy in the diet, furnishing twice the calories of carbohydrates or protein per gram. Fat provides 9 calories per gram.

The components of fats are saturated or unsaturated. Saturated fatty acids are generally solid at room temperature and derived primarily from animal sources.

Unsaturated fatty acids are usually liquids and come from vegetables, fish, nuts, or seed sources.

Fats assist in making food tastier and increase satiety. Around 25% percent of your daily food intake should come from fat. *Fats should not be avoided*, only limit intake of saturated fats, such as high-fat meats, full-fat dairy, and packaged products. Aim for four grams per serving or less when choosing packaged foods that contain saturated fats.

Choose healthy options, such as unsaturated and polyunsaturated fats, which include omega-3 and omega-6.

Monounsaturated	Polyunsaturated	Saturated	Trans Fat
Olive oil	Fatty fish like salmon, shellfish	Animal source	Processed foods
Avocado	Walnut	Red meat	Fried foods
Nuts	Flaxseed	Dairy Products	Partial hydrogenated
Lower LDL	Lower LDL	Coconut oil, palm oil	Processed foods
Increase HDL	Increase HDL	Decrease HDL / increase LDL	Decrease HDL/ increase LDL

Trans Fats

Trans fats are fats that have been manufactured to increase shelf life and make fat harder at room temperature. The process makes crackers and cookies crispier. Trans fats are found in restaurant and packaged foods. Trans fats will increase your blood cholesterol, thereby increasing risk for heart disease and heart attack.

Vitamins

The vitamins available to us by eating a variety of foods include A, K, E, D, B, and C. Vitamins A, K, E, D are fat-soluble. This means fat is required for vitamin absorption and storage. Vitamins B and C are water-soluble, which are excreted through the kidney when taken in higher amounts than body needs

In order for your body to produce collagen, you need vitamin C. Collagen provides structure in bone, blood vessels, and ligaments. Rich sources include strawberries; oranges, lemons, limes, and other citrus; kiwi and peppers. Vitamin D regulates blood-calcium levels and calcium absorption in bones. Vitamin D is found in food sources like fortified cereal and dairy products. Certain fatty fish, like cod, herring, oysters, halibut, salmon, and sardines, contain vitamin D. Your body can make vitamin D after sunlight exposure.

Minerals

Our bodies cannot synthesize minerals; therefore, we must consume them daily. Certain fad diets will not include the variety of nutrients the body requires to function efficiently— this is the reason for eating a variety of foods and not restricting a particular nutrient.

Minerals provide structure in forming and maintaining teeth and bones. Also, minerals play a major role in keeping a normal heart rhythm, muscle contraction, and healthy nervous system.

The difference between major and trace minerals are the amount needed daily. Trace minerals are zinc, iron, copper, selenium, iodine, fluorine, and chromium. Daily intake requirement are less than 100 mg per day.

Major minerals are calcium, sodium, potassium, phosphorus, magnesium, manganese, sulfur, chlorine, and cobalt. Daily intake requirement is more than 100 mg per day. Fish, dairy products, and dark-green leafy vegetables contain minerals.

Water

Water helps transport nutrients into cells and maintains homeostasis in the body. When you fail to replenish the water your body needs, it will retain the limited amount of water it has, along with retaining fat. The liver is the organ that deals with breaking down fat, and kidneys deal with filtering toxins. If you do not have enough water in your system, your kidneys will not be able to do their job, and your body will shift some of the work back to the liver. The liver, which was dealing with breaking down fat, now has to also deal with filtering what the kidneys would normally be doing. This compromises the liver's efficiency and winds up leaving most of the fat in your body that it would normally burn.

Headaches, lack of ability to concentrate, muscle cramps, increased blood pressure, decreased and dark urine, tiredness, irritability, and nervousness are symptoms of dehydration. How ironic—these symptoms are usually attributed to hunger.

You may be dehydrated and not even know it. Initially, you may experience thirst, but for many, the "thirst signal" is confused with the "hunger signal."

When dehydrated, you will appear heavier on the scale because your body will bloat—this is a sure sign of dehydration.

8

Checklist

Practice daily and focus on at least two strategies:
Antecedent ☐
Behavior ☐
Consequence ☐
Drink water before your shower. ☐
Drink water after your shower. ☐
Drink water before your meal. ☐
Drink water after your meal. ☐
Eat slowly. ☐
Read labels. ☐
Know your serving size. ☐
Cut out regular or diet soda. ☐
Cut out fruit juices. ☐
Identify your triggers. ☐
1.
2.
3.
Modify your triggers. ☐
1.
2.
3.

Do a three minute cardio activity in the morning to boost energy. □

Hold in your abs while sitting at your desk, driving, watching television, waiting in line. □

9

Helpful Hints

Having a well-stocked pantry makes cooking doable anytime. Start with the items that appeal to you. Substitute frozen if you don't have fresh items on hand. Use herbs to spice things up.

A list of items that is necessary to have in your freezer, fridge, and pantry includes the following:

Poultry	Frozen spinach	Dried oregano
Turkey slices	Frozen broccoli	Curry powder
Turkey hamburgers	Frozen cauliflower	Dried thyme
Turkey Sausage	Frozen mixed peppers	Dried dill
Unsalted nuts (almonds, walnuts, etc.)	Onions	Cayenne
Almond butter	Garlic	Paprika
Peanut butter	Canned tomatoes (diced, whole or chopped).	Garlic powder

Eggs	Mushrooms in jar	Cumin, rosemary, thyme, basil
Quinoa	nonstick cooking spray (variety of flavor)	Ginger
Ready-prepared salad	Flaxseed (seeds and ground)	High protein bread

- Most ingredients in a recipe may be substituted with another. For example, whole-wheat bread crumbs for coating is preferred, but you can substitute Panko or other breadcrumbs you have available.
- Adjust recipes to your taste. Use less or more seasoning and herbs. This is an individual preference.
- Double the amount of the sour cream recipe (see "Recipes," chapter 11) used for the asparagus, and use on any other vegetable you desire.
- Substitute vegetables according to what you like and what is in season.
- Regular and 2% milk have about the same fat content. Always go for 1% or fat-free.

- Always have cooking spray on hand and use when sautéing. It keeps food from sticking since a small amount of olive oil is used.
- Store bought ground turkey can have about the same amount of fat (or worse if you use lean beef). Best ground turkey to purchase is *85lean/15fat or 90 lean /10fat.*
- If you don't have an electric griller, I suggest you invest in one.
- A few of the many ideas for including flaxseed in your daily meal plan are:
  - ➤ Add flaxseed to marinades.
  - ➤ Sprinkle ¼-teaspoon ground flaxseed onto salad, yogurt, and vegetables.
  - ➤ Include flaxseed in your salad dressing mix.
  - ➤ Use flaxseed in baking or add to hamburger, meatloaf, or other similar dishes.

10

Meal Plans

Meal plans facilitate strategies, and you will find your eating habits remain even after you are off the plan. Stick to this meal plan for two weeks. If you have more weight to lose, go back and repeat. However. This time you can substitute nutrients. For example, instead of having fish, opt for egg whites, turkey, or chicken. Change up the greens.

Recipes for foods listed in italics are given in chapter 11.

Breakfast
Asparagus and Mushroom Quiche
or
Easy Eggs

Snack
1/4 cup raw almonds
or
Greek yogurt (non-fat, any flavor), plus 2 tablespoon *savory nuts*

Lunch
5 ounces easy tuna
8–12 asparagus stalks, steamed or grilled

Snack
1 cup summer yogurt
or
¾ cup Greek yogurt, non-fat
1/8 cup of savory nuts

Dinner
Easy salmon
or
Halibut with Green Beans and Tomato
or
6–8 ounces fish (any variety)
1–2 cups of steamed broccoli

Bedtime Snack
Turkey Roll-Up
or
20 grams- protein shake

If you crave something sweet and fulfilling: 2 pieces of high-protein bread, one-ounce low-fat cheese, 1 tablespoon fig preserve. Grill on electric griller. The sweetness of the preserve along with the melted cheese satisfies any craving. Yet, it is fulfilling and healthy.

11

Recipes

You may not like to follow recipes or have a great deal of time to spend in the kitchen. The great news about the recipes in this chapter is they take very little time to prepare. You probably have most of the ingredients already. If you don't care for a certain spice or ingredient, you can substitute. The recipe will taste great regardless if you use a white or red onion. Should you decide to use a red pepper instead of green, the recipe will taste just as good. These simple, healthy dishes do not require much skill, fancy equipment, or exotic ingredients. It is everyday food, cooked at home by busy people like you and me.

Infused Water
Adding a bit of flavor to your water will encourage you to drink more. Use one or a variety of fruits or vegetables in your water. You can add orange, lemon, lime, kiwi, berries, cucumber, celery, or fresh mint in a pitcher or bottle of water.

Spiced Water
Wash and peel pineapple, leaving some pulp on the skin. Pour 64 ounces of water in a pot. Place pineapple skin in water, along with cinnamon or cloves (add according to your preference) or

both. Boil, and then cool to room temperature. It is delicious as well as a diuretic.

Cheese Mixture

In a Ziploc bag, 2 percent fat extra sharp shredded cheese or any variety, along with same amount of fat-free cheese (same type of cheese)—this cuts back on calories. It freezes well and can be used with any recipe that calls for cheese.

Savory nuts

6 cups of your favorite unsalted nuts
1 cup dried fruits, chopped (raisins, figs, dates, cranberry)
2-3 tablespoon cinnamon, grounded

Place nuts, dried fruit, and cinnamon in Ziploc bag, mix, and freeze. When you are in need of a quick snack measure out ½ cup and take with you. To make it a meal, add 1/8 cup savory nuts to 1 cup Vanilla non-fat Greek yogurt.

Pecan nuts are rich in calories and good fat. Yet, contains many health benefits and keep your hunger at bay.

Vegetables

Roasted Eggplant and Peppers

1 medium eggplant
1 medium red bell pepper
1 medium yellow bell pepper (any variety)
1 medium onion (any variety)
2 teaspoons extra-virgin olive oil
1/4 cup balsamic vinegar
1/4 cup rosemary, chopped, or 2 tablespoons dried rosemary
crushed pepper (optional)

In a Ziploc bag, mix olive oil, balsamic vinegar, rosemary, and crushed pepper. Wash and cut vegetables about a quarter inch wide, and place vegetables in the dressing mixture. Place marinated vegetables in the fridge until ready to bake. Marinating vegetables will decrease cook time and food will have more flavor. *This is a planning strategy to pre-prepare your meals ahead of time.* Although, you can use immediately.

Preheat oven to 450 degrees. Spray cookie sheet with olive oil spray. Place vegetables on cookie sheet. Spray vegetables with olive oil spray. Cook for 15–20 minutes. (The length of time will vary by the type and size of vegetable and your preference on tenderness.)

Easy Cabbage Slaw
1 medium head cabbage, shredded (red, white or both)
1 medium onion, diced
1 large red, green, or yellow pepper, sliced (use all three for an array of color and vitamins)
1 large tomato, chopped (optionaql)
1 large clove garlic, mashed
1 tablespoon extra-virgin olive oil
1/4 cup balsamic vinegar
1 teaspoon salt
1 tablespoon crushed pepper (optional)

In a covered container, place prepped vegetables. In a separate small bowl, whisk garlic, olive oil, balsamic vinegar and salt. Pour over cabbage mixture, close container, and mix by shaking container.

When I don't have time to prepare dressing, I use 1/8 cup light raspberry dressing for the entire recipe. It tastes just as good.

Cabbage keeps well in the refrigerator. A great strategy is to prepare and have enough for leftovers.

Cauliflower Delight

1 medium cauliflower head, cored and cut into bite-size florets, or frozen cauliflower (about 4 cups)
2 medium garlic cloves, chopped
1 tablespoon extra-virgin olive oil
3 tablespoons parmesan cheese
1/4 cup warm water
1/2 cup parsley, finely chopped
2 teaspoons brown pepper

In a large skillet over high heat, heat olive oil. Rinse cauliflower and leave wet. Add garlic to oil, and cook for 2 minutes, stirring frequently. Add cauliflower to garlic, and stir until it turns light brown. Add water, cover, and cook on medium for 8–10 minutes.

Once cauliflower is tender, turn off heat and add Parmesan, parsley, and brown pepper.

May be eaten hot or at room temperature. To intensify flavor, continue cooking on low to medium heat, uncovered, until liquid evaporates.

Great as a side dish or add protein and make it a complete meal.

Lemony Asparagus

2 pounds fresh asparagus
6 cups water
3 tablespoons seasoned Panko crumbs
3 tablespoons grated Parmesan cheese
1/3 cup fat-free sour cream
1 1/2 teaspoons grated lemon zest
2 1/2 tablespoons fresh lemon juice
1 teaspoon garlic powder
1 teaspoon extra-virgin olive oil
fat-free cooking spray

Preheat oven to 450 degrees. Bring water to boil in a saucepan. Add asparagus, and cook until crisp-tender, about 4 to 6 minutes. (Time can vary, according to your desired asparagus crispness.) Drain in colander.

Mix Panko and Parmesan in bowl. In a separate bowl, whisk sour cream, lemon zest, lemon juice, garlic powder, and olive oil.

Place asparagus on a cookie sheet sprayed with olive oil cooking spray. Spread sour cream mixture over asparagus and sprinkle Panko mixture on top.

Place under broiler for about 4 minutes until golden brown.

Tabouli

8 cups loosely packed parsley leaves, minced
1/2 cup fresh mint (optional)
3 scallions, finely chopped
1 large tomato, finely chopped
4 radishes, finely chopped
1/4 cup fresh lemon juice
2 tablespoons extra-virgin olive oil
1 teaspoon flaxseed, ground
salt and pepper to taste
romaine lettuce or cabbage

Use food processor to mince parsley or mince by hand. Lightly toss all ingredients except romaine lettuce or cabbage. Refrigerate until ready to eat. Place tabouli on a bed of romaine lettuce or cabbage leaf.

You can make this for your starter dish or add 1 cup cooked quinoa (cooled) to this recipe and make it your main meal.

Baba Ganoush

2 medium eggplants
1 tablespoon plain Greek yogurt (non-fat)

2–3 cloves garlic, smashed, with a pinch of salt
1/4 cup fresh lemon juice; more as needed
2 tablespoons parsley, chopped
salt, black pepper, and crushed pepper to taste

Preheat oven to 450. Wash, pierce, and place eggplant on oven rack. Bake for 20 minutes. Turn and bake for another 20 minutes. Cook until tender, charred, and skin appears black and blistered on all sides. Alternately, you can use the microwave to roast eggplant. Place in microwave and cook for about 5 minutes on each side.

Remove from oven and let cool. Cut in half and remove pulp. If some of the skin happens to mix with pulp, it gives the mixture more body and extra fiber. Add garlic, lemon juice, and black pepper to eggplant. Using a fork, mix all ingredients to the consistency you prefer. Sprinkle parsley on top of baba ganoush. Place in a tight container, and refrigerate until ready to eat.

If smoky flavor appeals to you, use 2 teaspoons liquid smoke to this recipe.

Blistered Broccoli
4 cups of frozen broccoli, or 1 head broccoli, cut into 16 pieces
1 tablespoon extra-virgin olive oil
nonstick spray
2 cloves garlic, sliced, or 2 teaspoons garlic powder (not garlic salt)
1/4 cup vegetable broth or water
1 tablespoon crushed red pepper flakes (optional)
1 tablespoon fresh ginger (optional)
½ cup frozen pepper and onion mixture (optional)
1 teaspoon flaxseed, ground or seed

Preheat large skillet over high heat. Spray with nonstick, and pour olive oil onto hot skillet. Place broccoli in skillet and char until broccoli blisters on both sides. Add broth or water, turn heat to medium, and cover. Cook to desired texture.

Use any other vegetable in season or frozen for the same recipe.

Cabbage Mixto
half a cabbage, thinly sliced
about 6 cups
3 cups of frozen pepper and onion mixture
2 cloves garlic, chopped
1 teaspoon cumin
1 teaspoon black pepper
1 teaspoon extra virgin olive oil

Place nonstick skillet over high heat. Spray with nonfat spray and add olive oil. Reduce heat to medium-high heat, and add frozen mixture and garlic. Once onion is translucent, add cumin, black pepper, and heat for about 3 minutes. Stir cabbage into the onion mixture and continue to cook over medium-high heat for 5 minutes. Decrease heat to medium, and cover for about 10–12 minutes. Stir frequently.

Substitute red cabbage for variety. You can eat this as a side dish, or add cooked ground turkey for a main course.

Zucchini Gazpacho with Basil
1/2 cup basil, chopped
2 medium green zucchini, sliced
2 medium cucumbers, sliced
4 scallions, chopped
1/3 cup lemon juice
1/2 cup Greek yogurt, plain (non-fat)
1 tablespoon extra-virgin olive oil

Blend zucchini, cucumbers, scallions, olive oil, and lemon juice in a blender. Add yogurt, and pulse. Add basil, salt, and pepper, and blend for about one minute. Texture varies to your preference.

Before your main meal, start with this filling, nutrient-dense, low-calorie cool starter.

Protein Meals

Quinoa Kebab

Makes approximately twenty quinoa kebabs
For filling
16 ounces turkey, ground (85/15*lean*)
1 medium onion, finely chopped
2 teaspoons extra-virgin olive oil
2 teaspoons allspice, ground
1 teaspoon cinnamon, ground
1 teaspoon black pepper
1 large egg white (whisked)

Quinoa Mixture
3 cups quinoa
6 cups water
1 1/2 tablespoons ground allspice
2 teaspoons cinnamon, ground
1 tablespoon black or brown pepper
1 tablespoon flaxseed or chia seed, ground

Place skillet over moderate heat, spray with olive oil and 2 teaspoons olive oil. Add onion, stirring occasionally, until lightly golden, 6–8 minutes. Add ground turkey, allspice, cinnamon, and black pepper. Stir and break up any lumps; cook until turkey is no longer pink and liquid is almost evaporated. About 8 minutes. Remove from heat.

Bring quinoa, spices, and water to a boil with the lid on. Turn heat to medium. Cook 8–10 minutes.

Remove from heat, and allow to sit with lid on. This can be prepared ahead of time; it's best used at room temperature. Preheat oven to 450.

Place all cooked ingredients in food processor. To hold ingredients together, add egg white. Use 1/4 cup to measure and make into kebab balls.

Place on greased cookie sheet and bake for about 20 minutes. Freeze leftovers.

Kafta

8 ounces lean ground beef
8 ounces ground turkey (85 lean/ 15 fat)
1/2 cup parsley, minced
1/2 cup onion, minced
1 tablespoon allspice, ground
1 teaspoon cumin, ground
1 teaspoon coriander, ground
1 teaspoon cinnamon, ground
1 teaspoon flaxseed, ground

Mix ingredients in food processor or by hand. Measure ¼ cup kafta and form in the shape of hot dog or hamburger. Barbeque or grill at moderate temperature.

This can be prepared ahead of time and frozen to be ready to cook. Taste great when grilled on electric griller.

Baked Kafta

Same recipe as Kafta
12 ounce can diced tomato in juice
3 cups vegetable or combination sliced eggplant, green pepper, sweet potato, zucchini
Preheat oven to 450 degree Fahrenheit

Place uncooked kafta in a casserole dish and add chopped vegetable of choice on top of the kafta mixture. Add the diced tomatoes, cover, and bake for about 30 minutes.

Chicken Burgers

2 pounds chicken breast, ground
1 medium onion, chopped
1 clove garlic, minced
1 celery stalk, minced
1/4 cup olives, chopped or sliced
1 tablespoon ginger, chopped
1/8 cup quinoa (not cooked)
1 egg white (whisked)
1 tablespoon sesame seeds, raw
1 tablespoon flaxseed, ground or seed
1 teaspoon salt
1 tablespoon pepper

In a medium bowl, combine all ingredients and place in a tight container or Ziploc bag. Place in the refrigerator for several hours or overnight. Shape into patties. Chicken burgers can be grilled, baked or barbequed.

Cooked or raw, leftovers can be frozen and used for a quick meal.

Turkey Roll-Up

8-1 ounce slice turkey (low-sodium)
4 slices cheese (low-fat, low-sodium)
½ cup fresh spinach

Place ½ slice of cheese and spinach on turkey slice and roll. Place turkey rolls in a tight container, and takes along for snack or your first meal of the day.

Substitute your favorite low-fat cheese and vegetable.

Bacon Wrap

1 package turkey bacon
1 can pineapple chunks (in water)

Cut turkey bacon strip in half. Wrap turkey bacon around one pineapple chunk, and use wooden toothpick to secure. Spray cookie sheet with cooking spray. Place turkey wraps on cookie sheet and bake in a 450–degree oven until golden brown. This will take about 10 minutes.

Take this to your next potluck.

Easy Tuna Salad

12 ounces water-packed tuna (albacore suggested)
1/4 cup onion, chopped
1 tablespoons red bell pepper, minced
1 tablespoon lemon or lime juice
2 teaspoons brown pepper
1/4 cup parsley, minced

Drain tuna. Using a fork, mix all ingredients, and refrigerate until needed. For a creamier consistency, add 1 tablespoons plain Greek yogurt, non-fat.

Use lettuce for wrapping tuna or use high protein bread to make a sandwich.

Ground Turkey Medley

16 ounces sausage turkey, ground
Half head of cabbage, chopped (6 cups)
1 medium sweet potato, cooked, diced
1 medium onion, sliced
1 medium green pepper, sliced
1 large tomato, diced
2 cloves garlic, minced
2 teaspoons extra-virgin olive oil

1 teaspoon brown pepper
1 tablespoon flax seed
1 tablespoon rosemary (spice you desire)

Place nonstick skillet over high heat. Spray with olive oil and 2 teaspoons extra-virgin olive oil. Add onion, garlic, and green pepper to skillet over medium-heat. Continue to stir and cook until tender. Add ground turkey sausage to skillet and continue to cook until sausage is no longer pink. Stir in sweet potato, tomato, brown pepper, flax seed, and rosemary. Add cabbage, cover, and cook till soft. You may need to add ¼ cup of warm water to the mixture to increase cooking time. This will take about 10-15 minutes.

Gingered Salmon with Bok Choy
1 tablespoon low-sodium soy sauce
2 tablespoons grated fresh ginger
Or 1 tablespoon ginger powder
1 1/2 teaspoons pure maple syrup
2 teaspoons seasoned rice vinegar
1 tablespoon olive oil
1 small shallot, minced
About ½ cup
2 heads of baby Bok choy, halved
1/2 teaspoon canola oil
2-6-ounce wild salmon filets
1 teaspoon black sesame seeds
2 teaspoons scallions, chopped

In a bowl, whisk soy sauce, ginger, maple syrup, and rice vinegar.

Heat olive oil in a large sauté pan over medium heat. Sauté shallots for 1 minute. Reduce heat to medium. Add Bok choy; cook for 2 minutes per side; transfer to a plate.

In same pan, heat canola oil over medium-high heat. Add salmon and half of soy ginger mixture. Cook fish for 4 minutes per side. Transfer to plate with Bok choy. Warm remaining soy-ginger mixture in pan over medium heat. Drizzle over salmon. Sprinkle with sesame seeds and scallions.

Easy Salmon

4- 6 ounces salmon steak
Garlic powder
Brown pepper
1 teaspoon flaxseed (ground)
1/8 cup low sodium soy sauce
1/8 cup of maple syrup

Sprinkle garlic powder, brown pepper and flaxseed over salmon steak. Rub soy sauce and maple syrup on salmon steak. Can be cooked immediately or place in refrigerator until ready to grill. Best to use electric griller.
Serve over cabbage salad.

Halibut with Green Beans and Tomato

4 (6-ounce) skinless halibut or cod filets
2 cups grape tomatoes, halved
6 ounces thin green beans, halved crosswise
Frozen beans may be substituted
2 tablespoons basil, coarsely chopped
1 tablespoon apple cider vinegar
2 tablespoons extra-virgin olive oil
1 tablespoon seafood seasoning (Old Bay)
2 teaspoons brown pepper

Combine tomatoes, green beans, basil, cider vinegar, 1 tablespoon olive oil, 1 teaspoon Old Bay, and brown pepper, in a medium bowl.

Heat remaining olive oil in a large nonstick skillet over medium-high heat. Season the halibut with the seafood seasoning. Cook until opaque throughout, 3 to 5 minutes per side.

Turn off heat. Add the tomato and green beans to the fish. Cover and let stand for about 3 minutes.

For variation, use chicken breasts instead of fish.

Savory Sausage

12 ounces smoked turkey sausage (kielbasa, lean), sliced ¼ inch
2 teaspoons extra-virgin olive oil
Nonstick cooking spray
1 small onion, thinly sliced
1 medium apples, cored and thinly sliced (any variety)
1 (16-ounce) jar sauerkraut, rinse and drained
1 tablespoon cider vinegar
1 teaspoon packed light brown sugar
1 teaspoon brown pepper
crushed pepper

Spray cooking oil in a large skillet and warm 1 teaspoon olive oil over medium heat. Add sausage and cook, stirring occasionally, until browned, about 8 minutes. Remove to a plate.

Warm remaining oil in same skillet over medium heat, and add onion. Cook and continue stirring until translucent, about 5 minutes. Stir in apples, cover, and cook until tender, about 4 minutes. You may need to add 1 tablespoon water to onion and apples to assist in cooking. Return sausage to skillet, along with sauerkraut, cider vinegar, brown sugar, brown pepper, and sautéed onions. Cover and cook on medium heat until liquid reduces by half.

To reduce sodium from turkey sausage, slice and rinse under cold water.

Easy Eggs

1 medium green zucchini, chopped
2 egg whites
1 whole egg
1 teaspoon extra-virgin olive oil
1 teaspoon flaxseed
1 teaspoon brown pepper
1 teaspoon dried oregano

Heat oil on medium heat, and add zucchini. Stir in zucchini and cook until tender. In a medium bowl, whisk eggs, flaxseed, brown pepper, and dried oregano. Turn heat to low-medium, and add egg mixture to zucchini. Continue to cook until eggs are fully cooked.

Prepare zucchini and place in a tight container for a fast breakfast or snack. Substitute yellow zucchini, or use both types when available.

Asparagus and Mushroom Quiche

1 teaspoon olive oil
1 pound asparagus spears, trimmed, cut into 1/4-inch pieces
1 medium onion, finally chopped
1 cup fresh mushrooms or 10-ounce jar
1 teaspoon fresh thyme leaves, chopped
½ teaspoon salt
2 large eggs
4 large egg whites
3 tablespoons fat-free milk
1/8 teaspoon black pepper
1/4 cup extra-sharp Cheddar cheese, shredded

Preheat oven to 350. Place nonstick skillet over high heat and add oil. Add asparagus and onion; cook, stirring, until crisp-tender, 5 minutes. Stir in mushrooms, thyme, and ¼ teaspoon salt. Cook; stir frequently until veggies soften, 6 minutes.

Coat six 4- or 6-ounce custard cups with nonstick spray.

Whisk eggs, egg whites, milk, pepper, and remaining salt in bowl. Add cooked vegetables to egg mixture, and whisk for one minute. Divide egg mixture among custard cups.

Sprinkle evenly with cheese. Place cups on baking sheet. Bake until edges are set and center is cooked through. This will take about 10 minutes. Cool on rack 5 minutes.

You can substitute broccoli, cauliflower or any other vegetable for asparagus. Freeze baked quiche, and when you have no time or for an option, take a couple on the road.

Italian Stuffed Chicken Breasts

6 -6-ounce skinless, boneless chicken breasts
1 cup of mozzarella cheese, shredded
1 cup tomato, diced
3 scallions, chopped
2 cloves garlic, minced
1 cup frozen spinach, thawed and drained
1 tablespoon black pepper
1 tablespoon basil, dried
6 scallion (green part only)
1/2 cup fat-free plain Greek yogurt
1 tablespoon paprika

Preheat oven to 450 Fahrenheit. Pound chicken breast and set aside. Mix cheese, tomatoes, scallions, garlic, spinach, pepper, and basil in a separate bowl. Spread filling evenly on chicken breasts. Roll each chicken breast, and secure with toothpicks, or tie chicken with green part of the scallion.

Place chicken roll-ups in a baking dish sprayed with cooking spray. Brush roll-ups with yogurt, and sprinkle paprika over the chicken. Cover and bake for 25 minutes. Once chicken is almost cooked, remove cover, and bake until golden brown for 5 minutes.

Use cheese mixture of half regular and half fat-free. Any variety of cheese can be used.

Sautéed Chicken

1 tablespoon extra-virgin olive oil
4-6 ounces chicken breast, boneless, skinless, cut in strips
1 large onion, sliced
2 cloves garlic, minced
2 tablespoons fresh thyme leaves, chopped
1/2 cup fat-free chicken broth
pinch of salt and black pepper
crushed pepper, to taste

Place skillet over high heat. Spray with nonstick spray and add olive oil. Reduce heat to medium. Add chicken breasts to skillet and Sauté for 4 minutes; turn chicken over and add sliced onion. Cover and cook for 5 minutes. Stir occasionally. Add garlic, thyme, and broth. Cover and cook until the onion is tender. Stir occasionally for 5 minutes. Season chicken with salt, brown pepper and crushed pepper.

Eggplant Lasagna

3 large eggplants, washed and slice into 1/8-inch diagonal or circle
1 medium sweet potato (partially cooked) (For sake of time, use microwave to cook)
1 pound turkey, ground
1 medium onion, chopped
1 medium pepper, chopped
3 cloves garlic, minced

2 teaspoons extra-virgin olive oil
1 cup mushrooms, sliced, or 1-10-ounce jar (rinsed and drained)
1 (28-ounce) can diced tomatoes (no salt)
1/4 cup fresh basil, or 1 tablespoon dried basil or oregano
Nonstick cooking spray, olive oil flavor
1 cup of sharp Cheddar cheese (cheese mixture, page 58)

Preheat oven to 450 degrees. Wash eggplant and slice 1/8 inch thick. Use nonstick cooking spray on cookie sheet, and spray eggplant, top and bottom, with cooking spray. Place in a single layer on cookie sheet. Bake for about 15-20 minutes.

Place non-stick skillet over high heat, spray with non-stick olive oil spray and 2 teaspoons olive oil. Reduce heat to medium heat; add onion and garlic and cook for about 5 minutes. Add turkey meat, and cook until no longer pink and liquid has evaporated. This will take about 10 minutes. Add mushrooms and cook for about 4 minutes. Once all ingredients are cooked well, add basil and diced tomatoes. Leave on medium for about 5 minutes.

Cut sweet potato in same shape as eggplant, 1/8 inch thick. Pour enough tomato sauce in casserole dish so eggplant doesn't stick to the bottom of the dish. Layer with eggplant, sweet potatoes, meat filling, and cheese. Do as many layers as you can with all of the ingredients. Cover and bake for 30 minutes.

Don't forget to leave skin on eggplant and sweet potato for texture and fiber.

Zucchini Lasagna

Instead of using eggplant, use yellow or green zucchini. For colorful lasagna, use both variety of zucchini.

Sloppy Joes

2 teaspoons extra-virgin olive oil
2 cups frozen onion and bell pepper strips

1 pound turkey, ground
1 pound turkey sausage, ground
1 tablespoon Worcestershire sauce
2 cloves garlic, minced
2 teaspoons paprika
2 teaspoons black or brown pepper
1 (15-ounce) can crushed tomatoes in thick puree
crushed pepper to taste

In a large nonstick skillet, warm 2 teaspoons olive oil over medium heat. Sauté onions and peppers until tender, about 5 or 6 minutes. Add turkey and turkey sausage to the onion mixture. Cook turkey meat until completely brown for about 7 minutes. Add Worcestershire, garlic, paprika, pepper, and sauté 2–3 minutes. Stir in tomatoes. Reduce heat to medium low and simmer, stirring, until thickened, about 5 minutes.

To make it heartier, rinse a can of black beans and add to the final cooking of the sloppy joe.

Quinoa-Stuffed Cabbage

1 pound turkey sausage, ground and cooked
1 cup cooked quinoa (follow direction on package)
¼ cup tomato sauce (low sodium)
1 tablespoon allspice, ground
2 teaspoons black pepper
8 large savoy cabbage leaves
2 cloves of garlic, chopped
1 (14.5-ounce) can petite diced tomatoes
1/8 cup fresh lemon juice
1/4 cup parsley, chopped

Preheat oven to 450 Fahrenheit. Combine ground sausage, quinoa, tomato sauce, allspice, and brown pepper in a medium bowl.

Divide quinoa mixture evenly and place in the center of the cabbage leaves,. Roll the leaves over the filling, folding in the sides of the leaves as you roll.

Combine the diced tomatoes, garlic, and 1 cup water in a casserole dish. Place rolls over diced tomatoes in casserole dish. Cover and cook until cabbage appears tender and cooked. This would take about 30 minutes.

When ready to serve, top with parsley and lemon.

Complex Carbohydrates

Sweet Potato

Wash and pierce a medium sweet potato several times. Place in a microwave for about 8 minutes. Rotate halfway and cook the other side until it feels tender to the touch. Leave potato uncut for about 10 minutes, as it will continue to cook.

Sweet potatoes are a healthy, filling, and easy snack when you are on the go. Added to other dishes will provide flavor, nutrients and satiety to your over-all meal. Be sure to wash it, so you can eat the skin. The skin of the potato has most of the fiber.

M'Juddarah

12 ounces brown lentils

1/4 cup brown rice

1/4 cup quinoa

1 cup onion, chopped

2 teaspoons salt

1 teaspoon flaxseed, ground

1 tablespoon ground allspice

1 teaspoon ground cinnamon

1 tablespoon brown pepper

1 tablespoon extra-virgin olive oil

5 quarts water

Over high heat, warm olive oil in 8-quart pot. Sauté onions, 3 to 4 minutes or until soft and lightly brown. Add water, lentils, rice, and quinoa in pot over high heat. Allow the mixture to boil, and stir every 3-4 minutes. Turn down heat to medium low. Add the rest of the spices. Constant stirring is required so mixture does not stick to the bottom of the pot. It will take about 50 minutes for mixture to thicken. Add hot water and continue to cook if lentils need more cooking. Remove M'juddarah from pot and place in casserole dish to let cool. Eat cold or at room temperature.

The summer yogurt salad (listed below) or cabbage salad is perfect garlic, tangy side dish.

Hummus Bites

2 (15-ounces) cans chickpeas/garbanzo beans
2 medium garlic cloves, mashed
1/8 cup plain non-fat Greek yogurt
2 teaspoons ground cumin
1 teaspoon salt
1 teaspoon paprika (optional)
2 Cucumbers (any variety)
2 lemons, juiced or 1/8 cup lemon juice
1/4 cup parsley, minced

Boil chickpeas for 4-5 minutes. Drain but do not discard liquid. Place chickpeas in food processor; blend until smooth and creamy in appearance. Add garlic to chickpea mixture and process for another minute. Add Greek yogurt, cumin, salt, and paprika, and pulse for 2 minutes. Add lemon juice and mix for another minute. You can add liquid for a creamier consistency. Chill in a covered container, or place 1 tablespoon of hummus on cucumber and garnish with parsley when ready to eat.

You can make hummus boats using celery stalk, green, red, or yellow pepper.

Summer Yogurt Salad

2 quarts Greek yogurt, plain non-fat
1 cup cucumbers, chopped (with skin)
1/4 cup fresh mint, minced, or 1 tablespoon dried oregano
1 clove garlic, mashed
1/8-teaspoon salt

Mix all ingredients by hand. You can adjust consistency by adding cold water. Chill before serving. Eat as a side dish or savory snack.

Leave skin on most fruits and vegetables to increase fiber intake in your day.

Arugula and Chickpea Salad

2 tablespoons lemon juice
1 tablespoon extra-virgin olive oil
½ teaspoon salt
2 teaspoons lemon zest
4 cups arugula
1 (15-ounces) can garbanzo beans, rinsed and drained
1 1/2 cup grape tomatoes, halved
1/2 cup Kalamata olives, chopped, (optional)
2 tablespoons chopped fresh basil
Brown pepper to taste

Boil garbanzo beans for about 4 minutes and drain. In a large bowl, whisk lemon juice, oil, salt, and zest until emulsified. Add chickpea to dressing. Add arugula, tomatoes, olives, and basil. Gently toss until evenly coated. Season to taste with brown pepper.

Eat as a main meal or side dish. Serving size for side dish is about 1 cup and 2 cups as your main meal.

Oatmeal on the Go

8 cups oatmeal, plain (uncooked)
¼ cup chia, ground
¼ cup cinnamon, ground

Place oatmeal, chia, and cinnamon in Ziploc bag and mix. Put a tablespoon in the container for future measuring. When ready to use, place 2 tablespoons of oatmeal mixture in a mug and fill with water. Place in microwave for 2 minutes, stir, and heat for another minute. Drink any time of the day.

Oatmeal provides soluble fiber, which decreases cholesterol and is great for preventing constipation. Chia and cinnamon reduces high cholesterol, reduce inflammation, and enhances cognitive performance.

Baklava

A high-calorie, high-fat Lebanese dessert modified to low fat, low-calorie.
16 sheets phyllo dough
1 cup walnuts, chopped (pecans, almonds, or both can be substituted)
1 tablespoon cinnamon
2 teaspoons ground chia seeds
1 tablespoon stevia

Savory nuts can be substituted in this recipe. Measure 1 cup and chop by hand or food processor.

Syrup

1/2 cup honey
1/2 cup water
1 teaspoon lemon
Nonstick cooking spray (butter flavor)

Preheat oven to 450 degrees. Cut phyllo dough in half. Combine nuts, chia, cinnamon, and stevia. Place 1 full tablespoon of mixture in the center of phyllo dough. Close end and wrap tightly. Grease a cookie sheet with butter-flavored cooking spray. Place rolls on cookie sheet. Before placing baklava in oven, spray generously with cooking spray. Cook until light-golden in color. This should take 10–15 minutes.

Meanwhile, place water and honey in a small pot and heat on low until mixture is well mixed. This should take 3-4 minutes. Turn off heat, add lemon, and keep on stove until ready to pour on baklava. Once you remove the baklava from oven, quickly pour syrup over baklava.

Printed in the United States
By Bookmasters